# PSYCHOANALYTIC SOCIAL WORK

# PSYCHOANALYTIC SOCIAL WORK
## Practice—foundations—methods

*Michael Gunter and
George Bruns*

With contributions from
Martin Feuling, Sylvia Künstler, Horst Nonnenmann,
Olaf Schmidt, and Joachim Staigle

Translation: Harriet Hasenclever

**KARNAC**

The translation was generously supported by a grant from Heidehofstiftung, Stuttgart, grant number 59033.02.1/2.11

First published in 2013 by
Karnac Books Ltd
118 Finchley Road
London NW3 5HT

British Library Cataloguing in Publication Data

A C.I.P. for this book is available from the British Library

ISBN-13: 978-1-78049-090-8

Typeset by V Publishing Solutions Pvt Ltd., Chennai, India

Printed in Great Britain

www.karnacbooks.com

*Dedicated to friend and teacher, Ernst Federn, the late pioneer of psychoanalytic social work*

# CONTENTS

# FOREWORD

*By Estela V Welldon*

### Psychoanalytic Social Work: Practice—Foundations—Methods

I am delighted and feel honoured to have been asked by Professor Michael Gunter and Professor George Bruns to write the foreword to his new book. I have known Michael for a number of years, mainly through the International Association for Forensic Therapy (of which he is a past President and I am Honorary Life President) and have always been impressed with his tremendous gift for modifying and developing traditional techniques for the psychodynamic treatment of children.

This new book *Psychoanalytic Social Work: Practice—Foundations—Methods* by Michael Gunter and George Bruns is full of wisdom and practical down to earth applications. Its subject is about the bridge between psychoanalysis and social work. It took me back to the 1960s when I came into contact with the new "milieu therapy" at the Menninger Clinic in the US and subsequently with the "therapeutic community" in the Henderson Hospital in England. This was created by Maxwell Jones, who founded and developed the concept not only of the therapeutic community but also of "social therapists". Within the therapeutic community culture the young social therapists were very effective in dealing with people who have psychopathic personality disorders.

I have always considered it of great importance to acknowledge and respect both internal and external worlds, especially in working with antisocial behaviours. Mental or emotional suffering is expressed through actions which superficially appear to be against society, but are actually against themselves; in other words, a degree of self-sabotage. Here it is very important to remember Winnicott's axiom, that an antisocial act implies hope.

It has always been the tendency to believe that social work mostly deals with the lower classes, whereas psychoanalysis belongs to the middle classes. This book manages effectively to end this prejudicial view and shows how the two approaches can work in synergy for all social groups.

Of central importance is the teaching and application of the use of transference and counter-transference phenomena. This allows the psychoanalytic social worker to understand the conscious *and* unconscious dimensions of an encounter with the client. I think that Chapter Four is particularly useful in the understanding of adolescence. As mentioned in the book, "psychoanalytic social work can also pursue the goal of winning the parents' cooperation via an understanding of their own neediness". A process of involving not only the patients but also their families is being created in order to understand the intricacies, conscious and unconscious, of all participants. Of importance is visiting the family in their own surroundings, which, according to the author, is often the only way to ensure parental cooperation. In doing so, the family's neediness is acknowledged and successfully dealt with. Teachers and all other professionals dealing with children are intrinsically involved in these processes and this book is highly relevant for them.

The book is full to the brim with illuminating clinical vignettes, which have much to offer in the way of learning. In addition a glossary is provided with all terms clearly explained.

This is not only a most important book but also a much needed one at a time when so-called "pure psychoanalysis" continues to be challenged despite the fact that psychoanalytic concepts and ideas have become popular and have been taken up by the media. We need to demonstrate the relevance and vital importance of applying and supplementing these psychoanalytic concepts in the different humanistic professions, including social work.

Anyone who works with emotional problems, in this particular case social workers, but also teachers and all professionals will find this book a most invaluable resource full with very relevant information and insight.

This volume will without doubt become the best companion for people working in the mental field to turn to when dealing with particularly difficult patients and families, especially with dynamic changes occurring during adolescence.

I very much welcome its very timely publication, which should be read not only by those in the field of children and adolescents but also by all clinicians in the mental health field.

# INTRODUCTION

This book represents the first systematic account of the theory and practice of psychoanalytic social work. For students and those entering the field of social work who are interested in psychoanalytic social work it offers an overview of the diverse fields of practice of psychoanalytic social work and combines this with a description of its history, relation to other areas of social work, and relevant psychoanalytical theories. We are convinced for this reason that both for students on degree courses and also for social workers and social education workers in further training the book offers an important contribution and fills a gap in this field. Equally, it addresses practising social workers, social educationalists, and psychiatrists or psychotherapists offering comprehensive insight into this particular form of social work for those working in centres for counselling or early intervention or in social paediatrics. We have taken pains to make descriptions as clear and approachable as possible so as also to reach those who may not be familiar with psychoanalytic concepts. We have therefore included a chapter outlining the psychoanalytic theories of particular relevance to social work. At the end of the book we have, in addition, included around twenty definitions of important psychoanalytic concepts. In these definitions the relevance for the practice of social work is taken into particular account. The book is rounded off with a contribution by colleagues in the Association for Psychoanalytic Social Work in Tübingen/Rottenburg (Germany) bringing the practice of psychoanalytic social work to life in the form of case studies. Although aware that the kind of care offered in psychoanalytic social work will have to be, as it were, reinvented in every single case around the specific mental-emotional and social problems of the client, and that the relationship between psychoanalytic social worker and client will always have a highly individual, unmistakable note of its own, we nonetheless hope in offering this book to provide practising social workers with helpful tools for their task.

*Tübingen/Bremen*
*Michael Gunter*
*George Bruns*

## CHAPTER ONE

# Social work and psychoanalytic social work

The term "psychoanalytic social work" links two disciplines of an apparently contradictory nature. "Psychoanalytic" refers to a methodical, reflective procedure for uncovering *unconscious* impulses, connections, and meanings in which the analyst refrains from active or direct interventions in the life of an analysand. So this method confines itself to helping analysands to recognise and understand the *unconscious* factors influencing their inner life and social interactions. This enables them to make decisions and act in ways that are more mature, independent, and less predominantly fashioned by the *unconscious*. Psychoanalysis is concerned with a person's *unconscious* inner world and with the confrontation of this inner world with external reality.

As it is usually understood, social work, by contrast, very much involves "stepping in" to regulate and help in the external world. It seeks to influence external reality at least as regards the crippling, external, and above all material situation of people who have landed in distress. The combination of psychoanalysis and social work is rare in Germany. There may well be many social workers and social pedagogues who are inspired by psychoanalytic ideas but an organisation of social work that takes psychoanalytic principles into consideration only exists in very few places. One example of organising social work on a psychoanalytic foundation is found in the Association for Psychoanalytic Social Work in Rottenburg and Tübingen, whose work is described in detail in Chapter Fifteen of this book.

Before embarking on an examination of what psychoanalytic social work is we feel it makes sense to give a brief outline of the spectrum of social work.

## Social work—areas, developments, trends

There is a fair degree of haziness about the term social work and no consensus on its definition so we would like to preface further thoughts with a few comments on the original conceptions and on the development the term has taken. This includes its latest redefinition, recently marked in Germany by the renaming of *Sozialarbeit* as *Soziale Arbeit* (a little linguistic shift which is hard, or even perhaps impossible, to translate into English) as the field of practice of a postulated science of social work (*Sozialarbeitswissenschaft*).

With *Soziale Arbeit* two main areas are covered, namely social work as it has developed from "a history of care for adults" (Schilling, 2005, pp. 17 ff.) and social pedagogy which has arisen from "a history of care for young people" (Schilling, 2005, pp. 59 ff.)

Discussions in academic circles see the current position of social work as much affected by the fact that the decades in which national resources were channelled into the social sector in a continuously growing quantity are obviously now over (cf., e.g., Butterwegge, 2005; Krüger & Zimmermann, 2005; Sorg, 2005). So what was an astonishing expansion in staffing in the area of social work is presumably a phenomenon of the past. There was a tenfold increase in the Federal Republic from 24,800 welfare workers in 1950 to 235,000 social workers and social pedagogues in 2003 (Amthor, 2005, p. 45).

*Nolens volens*, whether we welcome this or not, in view of the straitened finances of the present day, suggestions are being made on how to make the best out of limited means. Spatschek (2005) for instance speaks of a "professional modernisation" which would consist in making programmes available to clients encouraging activity—following, for instance, the Scandinavian path from "welfare to workfare". The social work of today, according to these ideas, needs to concern itself with the consequences of modernisation and will necessarily bear some postmodern traits. It is bound to suffer from ambivalence over whether to help or not to help, whether to support *Lebensweltorientierung*—orientation to the client's environment, or to economise, and whether to foster individual responsibility or to emphasise societal cohesion.

One solution is seen in systemic case management (Kleve, 2005). Another, in a rather different approach, is the propagation of the idea of working in the client's real-life social network which aims to mobilise the latent resources to be found there (Kruse, 2005). An example of this is eco-mapping or genogram work that traces forgotten social and family relationships which can be reactivated (Budde & Früchtel, 2005). And a further suggestion is to combine individual casework with orientation to other networks (Klawe, 2005).

A second important question is that of the scientific-academic status of social work studies. It is true that with the Europe-wide changeover in all university courses to the bachelor's and master's model there are hopes of recognition for social work studies as a fully-fledged academic discipline. Greater social recognition of social work might at long last meet the wishes of the professionals in the field as they have so far generally seen their work ranked below its true value. There is, however, a prevailing uncertainty over its scientific and theoretical base—is it a practical science, a science of social action, a hermeneutical or a normative science? Anything seems imaginable (Birgmeier, 2005; Schlittmaier, 2005).

The research activities of a discipline give an indication of its current fields of interest and pointers to future fields of work. At a congress of the Deutsche Gesellschaft für Soziale Arbeit (German Association for Social Work) (DGS) sixty-eight research projects were presented in twenty-seven workshops (Engelke, Maier, Steinert, Borrmann, & Spatschek, 2007). Fourteen workshops, that is very nearly half of them, were concerned with topics generally requiring the setting up and shaping of a longer-term relationship with clients as opposed to one-off or isolated technical aid measures.

The topics of these workshops ranged from "The Life of Older Women" through "Violence and Prevention", "Children in Nurseries", "Foster Families and Upbringing in Children's Homes", and "School Social Work", to the social-medical (severely ill patients, social psychiatry, addiction) and psychosocial themes ("Coping with Difficult Biographies"). This preponderance of relationship-based fields of activity points to what qualifications are required in the social work professions, namely those that train students to be able to take on long-term relationship work.

The question "Is there a theory or science of social work?" (Erler, 2007, pp. 115 ff.) is still debated. It is part of a debate on profession-alisation which is connected with the progressive fragmentation of the fields of practice, the relatively brief history of the profession as such, the various different historical origins, and the many theoretical approaches balancing uncertainly between a critical and a conformist stance (cf., e.g., Bielefelder Arbeitsgruppe 8, pp. 147 ff.; Heite, 2008; May, 2008, pp. 69 ff.).

It is helpful in this general discussion to focus on the fields of prac-tice of social work and the methods used there. Discussing the major fields of work, Chassé and von Wensierski (2004) talk first about work with children and young people, covering a wide spectrum from early intervention, nursery school, culture, school, and juvenile court work, to work in parenting and family support, care of old people, support of women and the women's movement, and questions of disadvantage and poverty in the social state. They also describe a number of special-ised areas: sexual counselling, social work in the health system, social psychiatry, drug addiction, and migration.

Galuske (1998) describes nineteen methods in social work, among which are social pedagogic counselling, multi-perspective case work, case management, mediation, reconstructive social pedagogy, family therapy, theme-centred interaction, empowerment, street work, orien-tation to environment, also known as person-in-environment-perspec-tive, and supervision and planning of young people's services. Here the range of methods covers a great variety of approaches, marked by distinct contrasts.

As regards work with the clients there seem to be two prevailing ten-dencies: 1. towards an indirect form of work with them in which they are regarded as part of a network which is given the task of finding a solu-tion, and 2. towards keeping support as short-term as possible where the professional is regarded as merely providing the initial impulse for the client's own activities and for those of his network. Both may easily be combined with the systemic thinking which has become widespread in social work over the last ten years. *Sozialraumorientierung* (Früchtel, Budde, & Cyprian, 2007)—orientation to environment—with its SONI formula (social structure, organisation, network, individual) seeks to combine the two, naming four strategic points for the application of social work intervention. Working with this approach, it is not a question of offering technical aid, for instance an aid plan orientated to "the ideal of a good citizen" (p. 18), neither is it about a "psychosocial diagnosis" (ibid). The aim is to make the most of opportunities and situations. The hope is that changes will arise from a "situation analysis", intended to trace "situational potential" and lead to "situative efficacy" (p. 21). One outcome of the person-in-environment-perspective is intended to be the discovery and, if need be, the creation of contexts and contact structures (p. 25) out of which new situations and opportunities can emerge. The example given, as illustration, is of a guard dog which does not bark and so fails in its task. Its situational potential could be exploited with a warning sign: "Beware of silent dog!" (p. 22). Paradoxical intentions of this kind, however, presuppose the presence of reasonably well-functioning social and/or interpersonal systems if any systemic interventions are to become effective.

In more than just a few cases, however, there is no longer any functioning system available to clients, either of family or of friendship or even of a professional-governmental kind. Little Kevin from Bremen (Mäurer, 2006) is a case in point: he and his drug-addicted stepfather were well known to the social services but he did not receive help from the social services or from the neighbourhood or from any family circle that might have saved him from lethal abuse by his stepfather.

## On the relation between social work and therapy

A number of factors have led to an increasing use of methods adapted from therapy in social work and social pedagogy: one, as mentioned above, is the number of clients who lack any kind of social resource; a second, as Galuske (2007, p. 132) points out, is the 1970s critique of methods in social work; and a third, we feel, is the expansion of the areas of social work practice since the 1970s when a turn to psychosocial thinking emerged following the establishment of a new Medical Licensure Act (*Approbationsordnung*) which covered the syllabus and qualifications for doctors of medicine. This was also the period when social therapeutic institutions were planned as an alternative to prison sentences and when socio-psychiatric ideas and structures became prevalent.

However, with the adoption of therapeutic methods, social work is in danger of losing touch with the everyday world and the social environment of its clients, for therapy is always carried out in a special space set apart from everyday life. The classic field of social work is giving aid to people in need as a result of outward circumstances whereas the focus of therapy is people's inner state of need, their suffering through their mental and emotional disorders, and in simply being who they are.

Galuske is not wrong to emphasise the differences between social work and therapy (pp. 136 ff.).

On the one hand you have the great complexity of social work orientation to the client's everyday world and environment; on the other, the centring of therapy on specific areas such as perception, communication, emotion, and self-control; or again on the one hand there is the direct action taken by social pedagogue and social worker in the client's everyday concerns, and on the other the quiet of therapeutic "action" in a situation apart from the everyday; in the one field there are the social work interventions targeted to current visible, tangible everyday problems, and in the other the far-from-everyday interventions of therapy tied to a specific setting.

And there is the contrast between the clients of social work with everyday problems and interests in receiving social support and tending on the whole to belong to the lower classes, as opposed to patients in therapy with mental and emotional problems and a tendency to belong to the middle classes. In actual fact, in practice, many patients who are also clients of social aid systems benefit greatly from therapy so that we cannot agree to this last distinction which seems to wish to reserve access to therapy largely to the middle classes. Galuske is right that it makes sense to differentiate between social work and therapy—although above all in work with children and adolescents it is hard to see where the line between social pedagogic interventions, measures to foster development, and therapeutic interventions can be drawn (cf. Chapter Five). A further crucial difference can be added to those identified by Galuske, namely that the suffering which is the precondition for therapy is inner mental-emotional disorder, whereas the source of the suffering which is the precondition for social work is the outward circumstance of privation.

While it is true that both can be present, requiring effort from both systems of support, yet material want alone will seldom produce mental-emotional illness except in the case of traumatic experiences. On the other hand mental-emotional illness can well bring on serious material distress. In this case, too, both social work and therapeutic effort are required. In our view the perception of social work as shown in Galuske's analysis restricts it too much to material living conditions. There is a long-established and recognised connection between pauperism (in the sense of institutionalised poverty, poverty over a person's whole life and in some cases over generations) and mental-emotional illness. Mental-emotional suffering, as we see it, is one of the important areas of concern for social work.

As already mentioned in the examination of research topics, the methods and areas of practice which are increasingly coming to the fore are those which demand work on and with the relationship to the clients. This is reflected in the corresponding publications. Schaub (2007) describes theories, methods, and areas of practice of clinical social work, Denner (2008) social work with children with mental-emotional disorders, Kuhles (2007) social pedagogical "ways out of isolation" for autistic children and adolescents. Ortmann and Röh (2008), too, have edited a collection of essays on clinical social work, Lützenkirchen (2008) writes on social work concerned with depression in old age, Speck (2007) on school social work.

Work in and through relationships forms an important part of the various approaches in the publications mentioned and is clearly, as in Schaub's writing, informed partly by psychoanalytic concepts but, in addition, there are also a number of publications which are explicitly concerned with the relation between psychoanalysis and social work. May (2008) devoted a chapter to psychoanalytic social work in his book on current theoretical social work discourses. He did not however mention any of the many publications from the members of the Association for Psychoanalytic Social Work in Tübingen, nor Stemmer-Lück's book (2004) on "Spaces for Relationships in Social Work" which is exclusively concerned with the relationship between psychoanalysis and social work and the possibility of using psychoanalytic theories in social work. One special issue of the journal *Kinderanalyse* entitled "Psychoanalytic Social Work" (no. 1/14:2006) outlines the subject of psychoanalytic social work in a series of contributions (August Aichhorn, 2006; Thomas Aichhorn, 2006; Bruns, 2006; Feuling, 2006; Gunter 2006a). We see all these publications as pointing to a growing need in social work for an approach such as those which psychoanalysis and its perceptions can offer to the problems that emerge in work with clients, an approach needing and using the relationship with the client. Psychoanalytic social work is an application of psychoanalysis in the social area and this is one of the three major areas of its application alongside the clinical and the cultural. Its application is appropriate when in addition to an external situation of destitution or neediness there is a serious mental-emotional or interactional disorder, in other words in a doubly problem-laden combination of outer and inner need which cannot be overcome with the use of technical-instrumental forms of aid alone. It can be performed by all professions in the psychosocial field—social workers, social pedagogues, psychologists, doctors, teachers, nurses, and others. Psychoanalytic social work combines instrumental help with the deliberate use of the relationship to the client. *Using* the relationship refers to being aware of latent and *unconscious* elements in the relationship, regarding them as non-verbal statements about the client and the intersubjective combination. *Using* also refers to taking these into consideration in the planning of help to be offered. At the visible level, relationship is seen as meaning the committed character of a contact, communication, and understanding. At a latent and partly *unconscious* level, relationship means giving the other person significance.

To allow oneself to be involved in this way in a relationship is no easy thing, for we often sense intuitively very early on in a contact whether the relationship with this person is going to be fairly easy or whether it is likely to become complicated, burdensome, and taxing.

We often have a spontaneous defensive reaction to a relationship that could become complicated and demanding with the result that we avoid entering the relationship altogether. This can easily happen particularly with patients or clients who suffer from narcissistic disorders because they almost always have a pathological manner of shaping relationships. Some therapy concepts in the psychosocial area, such as the therapeutic chain in social psychiatry, have developed from therapists' unconscious wish to protect themselves from taxing relationships (Bruns, 1998). In the *therapeutic chain* as soon as patients have developed a relationship for a certain time and are feeling better they are moved on to the next station in the chain. In this way the difficult and burdensome aspects of the relationship are not worked on. This practice, like a number of others, represents a form of institutionalised *defence* against relationship.

The element of setting up and *using* a relationship in work with clients makes it clear that psychoanalytic social work is hardly likely to be attempted if only brief, one-off contacts with clients take place.

It requires a setting in which help or support is offered for a medium or longer period of time. Two examples follow.

## The long-term care of an adolescent

Bob is a member of the group in a group home run by the association Verein für Psychoanalytische Sozialarbeit in Rottenburg und Tübingen (see Nonnenmann 2003, pp. 136 ff.) and joined the group as a schoolboy. He was born in the Philippines, apparently in circumstances of extreme destitution. He is said to have fed himself already as a very small child on what he could find on waste dumps because there was nothing else to be had. At the age of two and a half he was adopted by a German family, in which there were two other, older adopted children. After what was at first a rapid development in which he made good many deficits in his earlier development, learning inhibitions began to emerge at school. He switched to a Waldorf (Rudolf Steiner) day and boarding school. At some stage he began to take drugs and smoke hashish regularly. He suffered anxieties, sleep disorders, ideas of suicide, and the conviction that the others wanted him removed from this school. He was committed to a psychiatric clinic for adolescents, referring to his own state as dope-head psychosis. After he was discharged from the clinic he entered the group home.

There he showed a highly developed sensitivity to the weaknesses and vulnerabilities of the staff and members of the group, exploiting these to torment them or get them to do things for him. At the same time he showed a great need for closeness and contact, seeking this from the staff. However, as soon as he gained the attention which did him good he would switch abruptly to making scathing remarks and using denigrating language. Things came to a climax when the wounding remarks he made and troublesome scenes he created became increasingly intolerable. Finally he was told he had reached the limit the staff could tolerate. He reacted with an overdose of psychotropic drugs leading to his being committed to a psychiatric clinic. When his state improved he returned to the group home but again was unable to fit in and get on even tolerably with the others. The attempt to allow him to live on his own in a guest house failed. He developed a paranoid psychosis requiring treatment in a psychiatric acute case ward. Finally after a longer period he returned to the group home and now for the first time began to think seriously about whether he really wanted to stay in the home.

There are many indications from empirical investigations and also from clinical observations and experiences that a fundamental, life-threatening rejection or neglect of a child in his first year forms one of the major risk factors for the development of a psychosis in later life. On the basis of this experience one is justified in regarding his parents' apparently total neglect of Bob in his early childhood as the cause of his psychotic episodes. He had experienced genuinely destructive hostility in his early *object relations* if we assume that for a small child neglect is also a form of abuse. But Bob's experience with his early *objects* was not only that they neglected him. They also failed to keep up any relationship with him. His parents' giving him up for adoption was probably not the first indication of scant or non-existent *object* constancy. We are probably justified in assuming that before this he had also been through very stressful and perhaps traumatic experiences of the breaking of attachments.

In the adopting family and in the group home he turns himself into the intolerable child to test whether people really want to have him or whether they will give him away if things get too difficult—so proving that they do not love him. In this staged narcissistic conflict his adoptive parents and the staff of the home group are substitute figures for the real parents on whom he unconsciously takes revenge when he overtaxes and torments his substitute parents.

The experience that despite the de-symbolised expressions of aggression and hatred in psychosis he is nevertheless able to return to the group home seems finally to have led to the beginning of a changed self-perception which challenges his self-concept of being a rejected person, so that he finally begins to reflect on his wish to stay in the group home. He no longer delegates this question to others, he now makes it his own. He no longer projects only hatred and rejection onto his entourage, a projection which had led to his paranoid symptoms. For various affects such as hatred and anger but also love he can increasingly regard himself as the actor. He no longer only sees himself as the object of other people's hatred, anger, or love. This is an enormous step from projective *defence* to the beginnings of taking over affects as his own and thus recognising them as belonging to him.

Bob is one of those adolescents with mental-emotional disorders who have fallen out of the safety-net of their social relationships and thus belongs to a client group which is important for psychoanalytic social work. Given the kind of disorder that these adolescents exhibit, given, moreover, the severity of these disorders which have led to their being impossible to care for by any of the usual institutions for the care of young people, and, finally, given the previous failure of the usual methods used in the care of young people, it is clear that psychoanalytic social work cannot confine itself to giving the impulse-to-start suggested by the systemic approach, which basically presupposes a client free from severe permanent disorders in his capacity for social relationships. We cannot turn to an activation of the client's network either because as a rule there *is* no functioning network to turn to, nor can it be a case of focussing on repairing deficits in material resources—as in classic care—because the cause of this serious psychic and social deviance is not material need.

Rather, psychoanalytic social work has to give very fundamental help to overcome the serious impairments in the client's social abilities, that is, above all, in the ability to relate to people, the ability to integrate socially, and the capacity for self-actualisation in social contexts. This also generally entails overcoming severe psychic impairments as a matter of priority. In the case of Bob and other adolescents, psychoanalytic social work is long-term care. It is a matter of several years. The work involves living with the person or persons in care during the social workers' working hours, and it requires the social workers to be willing to be involved in every client's intersubjective shaping of his relationship with them. It is based on two central elements: the instrumental work (material and technical help in the organisation of life) and the "emotional work" of the psychoanalytic social worker.

With this definition considerable similarities to another social profession are clear: this is the profession of the kindergarten *Erzieherin* (the title of which in German underlines the moral-social element of the work. She is literally an "upbringer " as opposed to the English nursery school or playschool *teacher*). Two essential differences are, however, to be emphasised: the *Erzieherin* deals with significantly younger children and generally works with relatively healthy children. By contrast, in psychoanalytic social work the work is predominantly with adolescents who already exhibit consolidations of their severe, mental-emotional disorders in their personality structure and corresponding pathological patterns in relationships. Nevertheless we feel it is worth noting how psychoanalytic social work definitely follows the tradition of social work as is found for instance in the institution known as *das Rauhe Haus* in Hamburg, where Ernst Wichern conceived social work as long-term communal living for clients with carers (Amthor, 2005; Schilling, 2005, p. 68).

## Medium-term help for an older woman

Frau F. is seventy-one years old, and was widowed a year ago. She has become something of a nuisance in the neighbourhood over the last few months. Dealings with her neighbours have become edgy since she first began showing unexplainable suspicion of them and then came out with obviously delusional-paranoid ideas. She claims people are saying bad things about her, that she is being harassed and that a man who lives a little further away keeps telephoning her with erotic intentions. She claims he hangs up as soon as she answers the phone. She has already written accusing letters to him demanding that he leave her in peace. The man's wife is puzzled and doesn't know what to think of the matter.

In her circle of acquaintances, confusion and tension have arisen. According to the information from the social psychiatric service responsible, a member of its staff has visited her and advised her to seek help at the socio-psychiatric counselling centre. In conversation with the doctor there it is perceptible that since the loss of her husband she has been feeling increasingly lonely and abandoned, despite still having social contacts. She misses both the familiar person to talk to and the feeling of having an exclusive understanding, and also an erotic bond with a person such as she had had with her husband. The doctor perceives that she has projected such feelings onto the man in her circle that she is accusing of making erotic phone calls to her. In warding off her wishes she has transformed them into an alleged harassment of herself: it is, at first, unclear whether these calls were ever made or were the creation of a sensory delusion. At the same time she has put a distance between herself and her moral self-condemnation for having these wishes by locating this condemnation in the minds of her neighbours. "People talking about her", which she imagines, and the everyday actions of her neighbours, which she perceives as chicanery, represent the punishment imposed by her *unconscious* moral notions.

Based on this understanding of the symptoms the doctor has regular conversations with her over a certain period of time and in these she can talk about her loss, about her past with her husband, and about her present feeling of being abandoned. After only two weeks she already reports that the calls from this man have stopped. Clearly she has very quickly established a relation to the doctor who has now become a significant *object* for her with whom she can talk about the hardship of her situation and what she wishes she had. In this way she can let go of the man in her circle whom she had turned into an imaginary partner following her *unconscious* but rejected wishes. Her phantasy that he was seeking erotic contact with her is something she can now give up. After a few more weeks she reports that the "gossip" and chicanery in the neighbourhood have ceased. As well as the conversations with the doctor, the member of staff who had visited her at her home informs the neighbours that she is receiving help from the socio-psychiatric service. At the counselling centre she joins a group of older women and men which is supervised by a social worker and she becomes a regular and lively member there.

In the case of this woman a paranoid syndrome in older age is not treated in a technical/instrumental manner with a neuroleptic, psychotropic drug, but instead is regarded as the expression of a process of increasing loneliness after the loss of a significant *object*. Accordingly the woman receives the offer of a helpful relationship in which she can present and partially realise her wish for relationship, exchange, and understanding. At the same time, corrective interventions are undertaken in the real world of the patient in informing the neighbourhood and in the extension of her social contacts with the help of a focus group.

## Relationship, emotion and development in psychoanalytic social work

The special and specific quality of psychoanalytic social work is long-term work with the relationships and the emotions both of the clients and the carers. In this it is close to the modern concept of psychoanalysis, according to which psychoanalysis is regarded as the reliving in the present of the patient's earlier, important relationships in the *transference/countertransference* relationship, which is the link between the conscious and the *unconscious*, with a new experience of relationship as the element triggering change.

As with general social work there are also differences and demarcations between psychoanalytic social work and psychoanalytic treatment. In contrast to psychoanalytic treatment, psychoanalytic social work has no formalised setting; it is not carried out in a "special space" in terms of time and place but forms a central element in the everyday world of the client over a longer or shorter period of time. Its tools are not word and interpretation but a broad arsenal of everyday forms of interaction—a glance leading to a word, a helping hand, and activities carried out together including physical contact. As regards the pathological processes of a patient the two main aims of psychoanalytic treatment are first, to make the *unconscious* conscious and expressible in words, and second, to achieve a partial, structural reorganisation. Of these it is only the second that is the specific and explicit aim of psychoanalytic social work.

The special aspect in work with adolescents is that they are generally still at a stage of volatile development which needs to be guided into a more benign direction.

Naturally, as with all clients of psychoanalytic social work, it is desirable that they should become more conscious of what they are doing as regards their actions, impulses, and staged dramas. But developing this consciousness systematically through interpretations, as in psychoanalytic *treatment*, is not part of day-to-day *care*: possibly if included as part of the complete care plan, this can be sought in additional psychotherapy which would be carried out outside the group home in a distinctly separate framework. Many young clients of psychoanalytic social work have only limited command of the ego functions which are important for communication, such as impulse control, the faculty of abstraction, and sublimation. The higher achievements of symbolisation, too, such as the use of language, writing, play, and the observance of rules are often only partially present because basic psychic functions of symbolisation and mentalisation were only ever fragmentarily formed. To foster and extend these faculties in the adolescent client becomes the central task of psychoanalytic social work. It can also be true for adult clients that where there is mental illness this is regularly accompanied by a temporary restriction of these mental-emotional functions through a frequently severe psychic regression.

Overcoming regressive states or deficits in development is often not possible without specialised psychotherapy. It is equally important that in their everyday lives the clients experience responses to their affective and impulsive utterances and actions that may be open and spontaneous but must not be naïve. By naïve we mean unreflecting and one-dimensional, that is without consideration of the context, the carer's state of mind, or the unspoken meaning of what the client has said or done. The considered response is only possible with at least a minimum of self-reflection. Of all situations it is in those which are charged with affect that self-reflection is most likely to be lost but it can be regained in the next step. One essential aid is given in supervision, that is talking over courses of action and processes with clients with an uninvolved third person. Supervision is not only devised to uncover unperceived interpersonal and institutional processes but is also a method of creating a reflective distance to one's own actions.

The effects of this reflective distance are probably felt in two ways: in the first, the psychoanalytic social worker can introduce a *triangulating* element into the situation by interacting with the client and simultaneously observing the interaction. This is a form of ego-splitting (Sterba, 1934) and it enables the psychoanalytic social worker to "take in" violent expressions of affect and respond with a modulated version of this input. In the second, the client can identify with this reflective attitude and with the transformed response. This process of transforming is, in Bion's language, the alpha function. If things go favourably not only the therapy itself but also the fostering of the client's development can lead to changes in the client's world of inner objects allowing greater differentiation through new identifications which enable him to integrate his affects and impulses more effectively.

## Preconditions for psychoanalytic social work

Psychoanalytic social work makes heavy demands on staff and depends on a number of preconditions. It cannot as a rule be an individual measure but is better placed in organised form in a small institution. Such institutions allow institutional flexibility which larger ones cannot; these always develop institutional dynamics of their own which disrupt or even destroy the sensitive, easily disturbed psychoanalytic atmosphere. The psychoanalytic atmosphere demands openness, patience, understanding, acceptance. Openness is required for the client's independent development: this means refraining from drawing up plans in advance which later have to be fulfilled. In place of plans what is needed is the readiness to allow unexpected developments. Often great patience is required to struggle for and achieve clarity and security in decisions: overcoming ambivalence to psychic change takes a lot of time and this has to be granted to the clients of psychoanalytic social work. They need time, too, to develop mental-emotional functions where they have deficits, such as in symbolisation and mentalisation. They need to come to an understanding of their conflicts, fears, deficits, and symptoms in order—via the understanding of the psychoanalytic social worker—to be able to understand themselves; what also require understanding are the frequently taxing and complex interactions which are often unconsciously designed to be complicated so as to conceal connections. Understanding is frequently only reached after long periods of time and until then incomprehensible behaviour has to be accepted. This is sensed by the clients as an acceptance of them as people, something of which many have had only rudimentary experience but which is immensely important for their self-esteem.

In addition to this, psychoanalytic social work requires a systematic reflection on the work done and this comes about particularly through supervision (Hechler, 2005; Verein für Psychoanalytische Sozialarbeit, 1994; cf. also Chapter Thirteen in this book). The aim of supervision in work with clients who have disorders of the severity discussed here is not only to offer expert counselling and correction but primarily to carry out detailed examination of the entangled interactions to which the social workers also contribute since they react to the way the clients communicate in a personal and very individual manner. Supervision then also becomes a place in which personal encounters can be talked over and it may be the starting point for further self-exploration. Because of the density of interpersonal processes in everyday living together, every social worker finds himself approaching the limits of his abilities to communicate appropriately and there is no doubt that a personal analysis is extremely helpful in these circumstances. Finally, supervision serves to stabilise the team of staff since with the kind of disorder the clients suffer from they will tend to externalise, act out their inner problems and conflicts in their environment. If this is not recognised then team members will take over various roles of the client's internal *objects* and find themselves carrying out these conflicts in external reality. Team *splittings* in psychiatric institutions are well known and are evidence of *unconscious* identifications with the inner objects of the patients (cf. Becker, 1995b).

Personal analysis—although to be recommended in psychoanalytic social work—is nevertheless a matter for the individual to decide on. Organised supervision which offers the possibility of reflection is, however, the responsibility of the institution which must make this possibility an integral part of the work. Regular supervision in the institution corresponds to the systematic analysis of the *countertransference* in individual psychoanalytic treatment, which is also often carried out within a framework of supervision or intervision. Supervision also prevents institutional *countertransference* reactions which may lead to the exclusion of a troublemaker from the institution or to making such a patient the scapegoat for the failures in the process.

## CHAPTER TWO

# On the history of social work and psychoanalytic social work

Today's forms of social work and social pedagogy have forerunners. These were arrangements for securing a livelihood for the weakest members of society through a political or social community which took over this task when—due to historical change in the forms of life and work—the primary groups of family, clans, and tribes, in which people had cared for each other, were no longer able to offer this support. A public system of care developed to secure people's livelihoods. This was imperfect and incomplete and for a long period it was intended to do hardly more than secure basic survival. Psychoanalytic social work is a more recent phenomenon, only possible after the development of psychoanalysis at the turn of the twentieth century and 1925 can be regarded as the year of its birth with the publication of two works: the books Sisyphus or the Limits of Education by Siegfried Bernfeld (1925) and Wayward Youth by August Aichhorn (1925).

## On the history of adult and youth care

The beginnings of adult care can be found in alms which represented the care for the poor of the Middle Ages. For youth care the roots are in the medieval care of foundlings and orphans (Erler, 2007; Schilling, 2005).

The care of the poor was to a great extent based on religious precepts. In the Christian doctrine of the Middle Ages poverty was given positive connotations. St. Thomas Aquinas with his doctrine of almsgiving gave a theological justification for the value and necessity for poverty. His view was that the giving of alms to the poor enabled rich sinners to do penance and so make amends for their sins.

At the beginning of the modern period, in the fourteenth to sixteenth centuries poverty and begging began to be valued differently. With the development of the capitalist economic system and the Protestant ethic that corresponded to it (Weber, 1905), work and the wealth acquired through work were seen as God-given. The poor were provided for if they earned their keep through work. New institutions grew up in the cities, prisons and workhouses taking in very different groups of social outsiders.

With increasing economic changes, particularly as a result of industrialisation in the eighteenth and nineteenth centuries, together with an enormous growth in population and the rise of the new capitalist economic system, the numbers of poor and needy multiplied, particularly in the towns, so that a system of care for the poor had to be developed. Whereas at first it had been a question of supporting the poor for work they were partly forced to do, in the nineteenth century the Prussian state laid the foundations for social laws under Bismarck's leadership. In the Middle Ages foundlings and orphans were put in the care of a godfather or guardian if there was one. In other cases they were housed in foundling hospitals or orphanages where the children mainly lived in miserable conditions. It was purely a matter of looking after their most basic material needs.

At the beginning of the modern era there were efforts made to set up schools for the poor and to have the children of beggars brought up by people other than their parents by housing them elsewhere. But these initiatives remained isolated rather than the norm. In the main orphans were housed in the usual places of care for the poor, that is in prisons and workhouses. At the end of the eighteenth century in Hamburg a new approach to reform of the poor developed in which child and youth care was separated from the general care for the poor and turned into a working education. Here a decisive influence was the system developed at the outset of the nineteenth century by Johann Hinrich Wichern in Hamburg in which children and adolescents were accommodated in small family-like groups in what was called *das Rauhe Haus*. The first steps towards a specific education for small children developed in the second half of the eighteenth century and first half of the nineteenth century. In this field it was Oberlin, Pestalozzi, Fliedner, and Fröbel (Schilling, 2005, pp. 68 ff.) who initiated what were to become the various forms of *kindergarten* and nursery school.

In Germany the beginnings of social work proper are commonly seen in the work of Alice Salomon who developed a regular training based on a "Girls and Women's Group for Social Assistance" in Berlin which led to a one-year course there for women in 1899. In 1906 it was extended to become a two-year course.

After the First World War, Prussia set up regulations for a women's profession in social work covering training with qualifying examinations, and introduced the professional title of "welfare carer". The women who graduated could then decide between "heath welfare", "youth welfare care", and "general welfare care". From 1933 the National Socialists made the training colleges form part of their *völkisch* ideas, such as "Women's Schools for the Welfare of the *Volk*" and introduced the title of *"Volkspflegerin"*.

After the end of the Nazi era these schools returned to and built on the framework established during the Weimar Republic, until 1959 when North Rhine-Westphalia carried out a fundamental reform extending studies to four years located in *"Höhere Fachschulen für Sozialarbeit"*— vocational colleges. From then on graduates bore the job title of social worker.

Alongside this training for women there were other factors in the development of the profession of social worker (Amthor, 2005). One in the Weimar period was a two-year training for men to be welfare carers. This was first started in the Seminary for Youth Welfare directed by Carl Mennicke, educationalist and theologian, at the Deutsche Hochschule für Politik in Berlin. Another factor was that significantly more men were trained in theological training colleges. Various Protestant schools for social welfare grew out of these initiatives; among others there was *das Rauhe Haus* near Hamburg. Similar institutions developed on the Catholic side under the aegis of Caritas.

On the Protestant side this training for men preceded that for the women's groups by many years. In 1833 Wichern had already set up a small children's home, *das Rauhe Haus*. Here care for the children was combined with vocational training. What was interesting in the organisation of this care was that it was founded on family groups. In these the "brothers", who were staff in training, lived together with the children. In the course of a four-year training to become a "house father" the brothers gradually took over increasing areas of responsibility in supervision, care, and training of the children. The aim of this complete immersion in the small community was not only the professional development but also the education in the person and character of the brothers. The training to be a house father was regarded as preparation for the tasks of director in Protestant children's homes. In 1871 there were seven *Brüderhäuser* with training courses for this male profession in social work.

The second main profession in the field of social work, that of the social pedagogue, also has a tradition built on various antecedents. The first was the *Jugendleiterin*, youth leader, and was originally purely a women's profession. The training for it received state regulation in 1911 in Prussia when the training to be *Kindergärtnerin*, or nursery school teacher, was also regulated. The first step to becoming a *Jugendleiterin was* to train as *a Kindergärtnerin* and after gaining relevant experience to take further courses at women's schools or appropriate lycées leading to a qualification for overseeing nursery schools, day nurseries, and institutions for youth care and education outside school hours.

In the period of the Weimar Republic their fields of activity spread, extending to running children's convalescent homes, seminaries for *Kindergärtnerinnen* and youth welfare offices. In the Third Reich the NSV, national socialist people's welfare, took over the *Jugendleiterin* training. In the early days of the Federal Republic training returned to the regulations of the Weimar period until in the midSixties the profession was abolished and replaced with that of social pedagogue, the training for which was then established at *Höhere Fachschulen für Sozialpädagogik*, specialist schools for this profession.

Only a few years later, at the end of the Sixties, these schools for social pedagogy and social work were transformed into colleges offering a training with a theoretical foundation yet orientated to its application in practice. The complete training was now four years with six theoretical and two practical semesters leading to the professional title of *Diplom-Sozialarbeiter* and *Diplom-Sozialpädagoge*. In various *Länder*, or states, the training to be a social worker or social pedagogue was carried out at colleges for both disciplines. From the overlap in the content what emerged was a growing similarity between the two courses of training.

Further changes in the orientation of content and organisation of these studies can be expected with the introduction of the bachelor's and master's courses in Europe, which according to the aspirations of representatives of social work will at last give to their studies the fully academic status of "social work science" (cf. Deutsche Gesellschaft für Sozialarbeit, 2005). This means that the term "social work" unites the training courses and professions of social worker and social pedagogue which have up to now been separate. The course of studies is to be established with bachelor's, master's, and doctorate so that at last academic posts can be filled with experts in the social work field and not, as now, with academics from neighbouring disciplines.

## On the history of psychoanalytic social work

Whereas social work with adults was and remained right into the twentieth century almost exclusively an undertaking to alleviate material need, the public and church provision for children and young people took on a different aspect from the beginning of the nineteenth century, namely the tasks of supervision, care, and education. The new professions emerging in this area were given titles that mirrored the task: *Kindergärtnerin*, *Erzieher* (educator), *Jugendleiter* (youth leader), *Sozialpädagoge*.

From an early point on, the educative intention of social pedagogic approaches, the desire to foster development, led logically to experiments in applying to the area of education and upbringing the new insights into child development which the emerging discipline of psychoanalysis was producing around the turn of the twentieth century.

A psychoanalytic education came into being. With *Sisyphus or the Limits of Education* published in 1925, Siegfried Bernfeld was established as the father of this movement. At this early stage in the development of psychoanalytic theory, Bernfeld mainly saw the psychological aspects of the drives when he writes: "[School] does not have an easy time of it. It is compelled to act counter to the children's inherited urges and against their spontaneous desires and interests. Whether methods are brutal or humane, it is forever in opposition to the powers of nature. To the child it represents the harshness and complexity of social reality with which mankind has been saddled ever since the Fall, whether it occurred in paradise or in the primal horde" (English translation by Frederic Lilge, 1973, p. 55).

According to Bernfeld's views the educator has to fight against strong aggressive tendencies, when he speaks of "the ancient sadism ... in whose shadow the school was first invented" (ibid., p. 55) and equally must struggle with the "goal-deflected love that drives him to 'his' children" (ibid., p. 103).

Bernfeld, however, also describes a relational field of many layers when he addresses the *transference* and *countertransference* relationship between educator and schoolchild:

> The child will love or hate the educator as it did the father or mother, or it will have a love-hate relationship with him ... What else can the educator do but accept the role thrust upon him whether or not he loves the child. He continues the parents' work albeit with other means, or he repeats it in a way that is new to the child: he works towards the destruction of the Oedipus complex even though the child's sexual love for him is not incest and its aggression not parricide. (Ibid., 1973, p. 107)

Here Bernfeld describes school in detail as a cultural institution demanding of children the renunciation of drives and confronting them for the first time with this demand on behalf of society—school education as the paradigm for culturally imposed renunciation as a decisive factor in the development of culture. This was the concept developed by Freud in the psychoanalytic theory of culture (1930a).

In addition to further articles on school (Werder & Wolff, 1974, vol. 2, pp. 5 ff.), Bernfeld also wrote on the psychoanalytic education of children, youth welfare, and education in institutions (Werder & Wolff, 1974, vol. 1). Soon after Bernfeld's Sisyphus book appeared, the Internationaler Psychoanalytischer Verlag in Vienna brought out the journal *Zeitschrift für Psychoanalytische Pädagogik* which was published for eleven years from 1926 to 1937. Then, when Austria came under the sway of the National Socialists, publication was stopped. In a collection of several essays published there, Weiß (1936) describes how teachers and pupils serve as *transference objects* for one another. Freud (1914 j), in a short contribution on the occasion of the fiftieth anniversary of the foundation of his old school, had referred to the *transference* significance of the teacher for the pupil:

> These men, not all of whom were in fact fathers themselves, became our substitute fathers. That was why, even though they were still quite young, they struck us as so mature and so unattainably adult. We transferred on to them the respect and expectations attaching to

> the omniscient father of our childhood, and we then began to treat
> them as we treated our fathers at home. (Freud, 1914 j, p. 244)

After the expulsion of psychoanalysis from Germany by the National
Socialists, for twenty years there were practically no publications on
psychoanalytic theory and philosophy of education in Germany. Hochheimer was the first to write on this subject again in 1959. He emphasised the way that children centre on the teacher with their needs and
how this encourages the stimulation of his narcissism. Fürstenau (1964),
too, stresses the central position of the teacher which could tempt him
to "satisfy a need for power without noticing it" (p. 75), but he also
discusses insights gained in the psychoanalytic theory and philosophy
of education of the Twenties and Thirties. These were insights into the
*transference* significance borne latently in the teacher-pupil relationship
and the suppressed warded-off drive tendencies in both teacher and
pupils (Bruns, 1994) which reappear in a number of school rituals.

In doing so he introduced psychoanalytic thought into the discussion on education which was just beginning in the Sixties in the Federal Republic. Not many years later these ideas spread far further with
the momentum of the student movement. Writings by representatives
of early psychoanalytic theory and philosophy of education, as for
instance Bernfeld, were rediscovered.

However, no new psychoanalytic education developed from this
new interest. The psychoanalysts hardly contributed to the discussion.
In *Psyche,* the leading psychoanalytic journal in the German-speaking
world, there were virtually no publications on this subject. Füchtner
(1978) lamented rather "the disappearance of a science and the consequences" (p. 193). He saw psychoanalysis as, on the one hand, marginalised in its increasing medicalisation and its orientation to medical
ways of thinking and preoccupations and, on the other hand, as merging into psychoanalytic socialisation research and child analysis, with
some motifs reappearing in the *Kinderladen* movement, the anti-author-
itarian alternative to kindergarten.

Finger-Trescher (2001), too, saw its medicalisation as a significant
cause of the disappearance of psychoanalytic education from psychoanalysis. Körner (1980) attempted to convince psychoanalysts of the
current relevance of the subject for psychoanalysis but received little
response.

In 1983 however, somewhat on the fringe of the psychoanalytic main-
stream, a grouping emerged concerning itself with psychoanalytically

based education which is still active: the Frankfurter Arbeitskreis für Psychoanalytische Pädagogik e.V. (www.fapp-frankfurt.de). It is run by teachers and social pedagogues who work with psychoanalysts and it offers psychoanalytic education in-service courses. The group has published two series of books, *Psychoanalytische Pädagogik*, running since 1990 and *Jahrbuch für Psychoanalytische Pädagogik*, since 1989. In the two series, the fundamentals of a psychoanalytic theory and philosophy of education are presented in which Trescher (1990) emphasises the importance of the teacher's *countertransference* and scenic, or enactive, understanding. Further areas examined are the possibilities of application, examples from practice, theoretical insights from other fields such as developmental psychology, social-political developments and their importance in a psychoanalytic education, and also the subject of school as a field of conflict (Büttner & Finger-Trescher ,1991). The field of teaching is shown to be potentially stressful to the point of cogenerating psychic disorders not only in pupils but also in teachers and a transgenerational passing on of such disorders to the children of teachers from the implicit educational mission to be a model (Bruns, 1989, 1991). The closeness of psychoanalytic education to social work is also documented in the publications of these series, for instance in contributions on "Psychoanalyse und soziale Arbeit" (Büttner, Finger-Trescher & Scherpner, 1990) or on the work of Bettelheim, Ekstein, and Federn (Kaufhold, 2001).

The beginnings of the other more care-orientated direction in psychoanalytic social work also date back to 1925. In his book *Wayward Youth* (1925) Aichhorn groups *"delinquent and dissocial"* with "so-called problem children and others suffering from neurotic symptoms" in the concept *neglected* (1983, p. 3).There was no very clear line between the first and the second. Aichhorn differentiates between latent delinquency, which he also calls a disposition to delinquency, and the manifest delinquency that is the expression of delinquency or symptom of delinquency (p. 41). He creates a classification of delinquency that parallels neurosis. Neurosis, too, may be present merely as a disposition in an unsolved neurotic conflict. It will become manifest in the form of neurotic symptoms when a person with such a disposition finds himself in a situation that triggers it.

So for him *Verwahrlosung* (delinquency) is a conspicuous form of behaviour in children and adolescents stemming from *unconscious* psychic conflicts in which, however, what is missing is "the quality of discomfort and unpleasantness which characterizes the neurotic symptom", and which makes "the neurotic aware of his illness" (p. 35). Like Bernfeld on the relationship between pupil and teacher, Aichhorn describes a *transference/countertransference* relationship for the relationship between pupil-in-care and educator (pp. 117 ff.).

He uses the *transference* for two purposes: first, it enables him to gather more accurate insight into the adolescent. In this way, as he describes it, "the transference in the dissocial child" regularly shows "a love life that has been disturbed in early childhood" (p. 119)—disturbed "by a lack of affection or undue amount of affection" (ibid.); second, he seeks to create a positive *transference* directly in order to have an atmosphere of willing cooperation. This understanding and cooperative way of dealing with "wayward" youths instead of applying discipline and repression was unusual at that time and opened up access to hidden causes of disorder. Above all, however, this new approach gave the adolescents the chance to discover and try new ways of behaving.

In Vienna a circle of psychoanalysts formed around Bernfeld, Aichhorn, and Anna Freud pursuing an interest in the application of psychoanalysis in the educational and social care area. They published their thoughts and reports on projects in the *Zeitschrift für Psychoanalytische Pädagogik*.

Fritz Redl was at that time a grammar school teacher. He took a training in psychoanalysis at the Vienna Psychoanalytical Institute and later directed educational counselling services in the city. The others, somewhat younger, were involved in their educational and social care professional training combining this with psychoanalytical training. This development of a psychoanalytic science of education and social work came to an abrupt close with the annexation of Austria by National Socialist Germany. Redl had already left for the USA in 1936, Ekstein fled there in 1938, Bettelheim and Ernst Federn were both interned in concentration camps and also emigrated to the USA after their unexpected release from the camps. There they were in a position to realise much that had probably already been planned in Vienna. Redl became professor for social work in Detroit where he built up the Pioneer House, an approved school for children from a slum in the city on which his book *Children who Hate* (Redl & Wineman, 1951) was based.

In the Fifties he was director of a children's ward near Washington which he organised according to the principles of milieu therapy he had developed with Bettelheim. Bettelheim, who had been able to emigrate to the USA in 1939, found a position at the University of Chicago where he was director of the Orthogenic School from 1944. There he treated mentally and emotionally severely disturbed children, particularly autistic children, with a milieu therapy approach. He not only published work on the treatment of psychically disturbed children but also on the necessary stimuli in the education and upbringing of healthy children *The Uses of Enchantment* (1976).

Ekstein, who had already studied psychology, philosophy, and history took a further course of studies in the USA in Boston at the School of Social Work to qualify as a social worker, and at the same time did a training in psychoanalysis. After that he worked for ten years at the Menninger Foundation in Topeka, Kansas and then for twenty years at Reiss Davis Child Study Center in Los Angeles where he worked with psychotic and autistic children and those with borderline syndrome.

Ernst Federn did not reach the USA until 1946 after being interned for seven years in the concentration camp at Buchenwald. In the USA he trained as a social worker and worked with juvenile delinquents and drug addicts. He returned to Austria in 1972 at the invitation of the then Federal Chancellor Bruno Kreisky and contributed to the reform of the penal system. With his assistance psychoanalytically based social therapeutic forms of work and supervision were introduced into the system.

Over their lives the psychoanalytic social workers and educators from Austria who built up an impressive body of work in the USA found there an environment for a kind of social work and a social pedagogic approach which did not exist in Europe. A form of social work focussed on the individual, with its starting point in psychiatry, had already developed in the USA in the 1930s.

It was a turning to the *subject* with psychological and particularly psychoanalytic forms of understanding. Important representatives of this casework were Florence Hollis and Gordon Hamilton. Following the perceptions of psychoanalysis, the client in question was to be enabled by intensive individual casework to tackle his own problems in an active and responsible way.

In this work the relationship between the social worker and client is regarded largely from a psychoanalytic perspective. Predominantly ego psychology interventions are applied and altogether this approach in American social work reveals a close connection to psychoanalysis (cf. Stemmer-Lück, 2004, pp. 4 ff.).

This early American casework approach differs, however, from psychoanalytic social work, as we understand it, in that it is far more or almost exclusively concentrated on individual cases, and interventions are used which are similar to those in clinical psychoanalysis. It is not orientated to milieu therapy or team-orientated work as is psychoanalytic social work according to our understanding of it.

In the meantime in Germany there has been a resurgence of psychoanalytic social work. In 1978 the Verein für Psychoanalytische Sozialarbeit e.V. was founded in Rottenburg and Tübingen, taking up the work of Ernst Federn and Rudolf Ekstein who regularly came there to supervise in the early years.

The association supports various complementary institutions in which adolescents are cared for who are suffering from severe mental and emotional illnesses and in some cases antisocial disorders. They live in group homes with carers, go to school as far as that is necessary, go through training for a trade, and receive psychiatric and/or psychotherapeutic treatment. It is a question mainly of adolescent clients who have been treated in psychiatric units or have already been placed in other institutions for the care of adolescents without having been able to settle down there. The intensive relationship-based work with them in which a psychoanalytic understanding of the disorders and interactions in the institution are worked through again and again in supervisions makes it possible in most cases to bring the negative career of even very severely disturbed young people to a close.

The association organises specialist conferences every two years in which members' work is presented and reflected on both in terms of psychoanalysis and of social work. The contributions to the conferences are documented in conference proceedings so that now a body of work filling many volumes has been collated, presenting the theoretical and practical aspects of psychoanalytic social work as it is practised in the institutions of this association. A more detailed depiction will be found in Chapter Fifteen of this volume. A number of other associations have since been set up in Germany and Switzerland on the model of the Verein für Psychoanalytische Sozialarbeit in Rottenburg and Tübingen.

CHAPTER THREE

# Psychoanalytic theories, methods, and concepts

Psychoanalysis as it is today can be seen as a complex discipline of different theories, concepts, methods, and of areas where it can be applied. As we view it from the standpoint of the sociology of science, it is appropriate to call it a discipline and not a theory. Though it is true that psychoanalysis developed on the basis of a "primal" theory, the psychoanalytic theory of drives, it has spread with the further development of the drive theory and the creation of new theories so that today—as in other scientific disciplines—there are theories which can be applied over a greater or lesser range.

Some theories contradict each other, presenting differing views of common concepts, and some concepts are very closely linked to only one theory. Wallerstein (1988), former president of the International Psychoanalytical Association (IPA), with his compact depiction of the pluralism of theoretical perspectives and culturally moulded forms prevailing in psychoanalysis today, has helped to establish a general recognition of the view that present-day psychoanalysis is a discipline with many theories.

What all psychoanalytic theories have in common is the assumption of the existence of the *unconscious* and its significance for human thinking, feeling, and acting.

## On methods and areas of application

The methods of psychoanalysis vary according to the area in which they are used. In clinical psychoanalysis, which is the foundation for all further applications, the clinical method of psychoanalytic treatment has remained as it was with the basic elements of technique being free association on the part of the analysand and free-floating attention and interpretation on the part of the analyst. There are of course modifications of the technique in the various clinical forms of application (low frequency or high frequency treatment, group analysis, psychoanalytic couple therapy, family therapy, and child analysis).

The interpretation, which refers to the current *unconscious* theme of the situation in the session, no longer arises primarily from the analyst's knowledge of *unconscious* processes but rather from his *countertransference* which enables a subtle perception of the psychic processes in the relationship between analyst and analysand.

The intersubjective, manifest, predominantly verbal and the latent, non-verbal communication between analysand and analyst becomes in this way the central process of a psychoanalytic treatment. Every psychoanalytic treatment becomes a completely individual non-reproducible encounter between two *subjects* each with his or her own ways of thinking and experiencing.

What is objectifiable and reproducible in this encounter are not the sequences in the process of the treatment or its results but the method of producing, shaping, and interpreting the encounter by the analyst. In psychoanalytic psychotherapy research instruments have been developed for the examination of the psychoanalytic process and its various parts.

The application of psychoanalysis to cultural theory differs here, based on the nature of the object. In the psychoanalytic examination and interpretation of a picture, of a literary work, of films, or of culture itself (Freud, 1930a) it is not a sensitive, acting, and reacting *subject* who exerts an impression on the psychoanalyst but an inert and therefore unchanging structure. This can be regarded as a frozen-in-time action or communication of the creator or artist targeting an anonymous recipient (Bruns, 1996), yet the work of art itself remains unimpressed and uninfluenced by the response or interpretation of the analyst-recipient whereas a patient in the analytic process reacts to interpretation with some kind of change. A work of art is thus not itself changed by a psychoanalytic interpretation. Nevertheless every analyst, like every other recipient, will make his individual interpretation of a cultural object in that he develops specific *transferences* and *countertransferences* to the communicative messages contained in the object (Pietzcker, 1992). In this way the effect of a work of art may be changed as it is closely connected to the way in which it is interpreted and understood. *Transference* and *countertransference* enable analysts to make their interpretations here, too, but they remain subjective since they receive no intersubjective communicative confirmation, negation, or adjustment as is received in the treatment process.

In terms of method, the third major area of application for psychoanalysis, the social area, lies between the clinical and the cultural. The psychoanalytic social worker, whether he or she be social worker proper, educator, or social psychiatrist, encounters a living *subject* as does the clinical psychoanalyst. He sets up a relationship with the client and uses his *countertransference* to understand the latent dimension of the encounter and the inner world of the client. He does not, however, encounter the other in the special psychoanalytic setting as the clinical psychoanalyst does (Stone, 1961). The encounter is in the everyday world.

It follows that the intervention instrument of the psychoanalyst in the clinical situation, namely interpretation, is not available. In psychoanalytic social work what is in the foreground is the relationship to the client and the enhanced perception through *countertransference* analysis of the way the client shapes this relationship. This relationship is also used to develop concepts for instrumental aid.

## Psychoanalytic theories

The major psychoanalytic theories are the drive theory, ego psychology, *object relations* psychology, self psychology, and a theory of intersubjectivity. In the following pages they will be briefly presented. Beyond that we offer an outline of the concept of mentalisation and of a few psychological aspects of puberty and adolescence since they are important for the understanding of disorders in adolescents with whom psychoanalytic social work is very much occupied.

With regard to the psychoanalytic theory of neurosis, Freud first assumed a traumatic origin of neurosis. But gradually he discovered the importance of unresolved psychic conflicts. Since 1896 he stressed psychic conflict as the source of neurosis. But he never revoked his theory of trauma, rather he assumed an interplay of *trauma and conflict* in the genesis of mental illness. His followers also referred to both although stressing more one side or the other. In general it seems that the more psychoanalysts treated narcissistic, borderline, and psychotic disorders the more they gave a particular significance to trauma.

## The drive theory

Psychoanalysis developed in a clinical context over the treatment of forms of hysteria known in the language of psychiatry today as dissociative disorders. The first publications on it were by Freud and Breuer in 1893 and 1895 (Freud & Breuer, 1895d). In the course of these treatments they discovered the effect of *unconscious* sexual impressions and phantasies as triggering hysterical symptoms, a subject which was then further pursued by Freud alone. These phantasies were initially interpreted as arising from premature or forbidden and thus traumatic sexual experiences. He extended the investigations to include other illnesses, the first being the anxiety neurosis (Freud, 1895b). Not many years later he published his early, major work "The Interpretation of Dreams" (1900a) in which, on the basis of his analysis of dreams he developed the fundamental principles of the workings of the *unconscious*, the influence of the *unconscious* on the conscious mind, the concept of dream-work as the process of reworking the latent dream-thought and concealing it in the manifest dream and the distinction between *primary* and *secondary processes*. Although Freud did not as yet use the term *drive* in these early works an implicit drive model underlies his constructions of psychic processes. This is particularly clear in his view of the anxiety neurosis which he regards as the result of a building-up of undischarged sexual tension with insufficient psychic processing. He introduced the drive concept itself in 1905 in "Three Essays on the Theory of Sexuality". With human sexuality as his model he saw the following as the four essential elements of the drive (1915c, pp. 121 ff.):

- its urgency, that is its inherent strength
- the source of the drive which is somatic in nature and manifests as a state of tension
- the aim of the drive which is satisfaction of the drive through release from the state of stimulus and tension

   – the *object* of the drive with which or through which the drive achieves its aim and which can be very variable.

Freud's drive theory underwent a number of transformations. He first of all set up a dualistic model of drive theory with two drives as the basis: ego drives or self preservation instincts on the one hand and the sexual drive with its internal energy, the *libido*, on the other. In his second, monistic model he assumed a unified drive fed by the libido which could, however, branch out into an aggressive and a sexual form, sexual in the broadest sense. His third drive model was again dualistic: this now, however, opposed the life drive to the death drive (1920g). With less emphasis on the derivation of the drive from an organic source the third model rather represented a philosophical attempt to describe order in living organisms.

   For the understanding of mental-emotional disorders an important element in drive theory is the concept of *partial drives*. Freud assumes that in psychosexual development, depending on the degree of maturity and in a characteristic sequence, different regions of the body become the most important source of pleasurable sensations, are charged with libido, and finally—in a normal development—come together under the primacy of the genital region, that is, governed by genital sexual arousal.

   The phases of development are an initial narcissistic phase in which the child makes no distinction between himself and the world around him. He regards the caring *object*, the carer, as a part of himself which satisfies his wishes and needs as soon as they are felt—a state from which the notion of the omnipotence of thought originates.

   This early narcissistic phase is followed by the oral phase with a focus of the experience of pleasure in oral sensations. The next phase is then the anal phase with a shifting of the predominant source of pleasure to anal stimuli. This again is followed by the phallic-narcissistic phase with a renewed shift of the most intensive sensation of pleasure now to the phallus or its equivalents, which may be a particular ambition or, particularly in girls, the person's own body.

   At each of these stages of development a fixation can arise through prohibitions, privations, and/or overstimulation, or through the impact of a traumatic event on the developmental stage, which can result in the predominance of the partial drive, a possible source of perverse developments. In the development of a neurosis, fixations also play an important part because, after the triggering of a regressive process in adult life, childhood points of fixation are again charged with libido and in this way determine the neurosis or the choice of symptom (see also Abraham, 1924).

The childhood psychosexual development comes to a provisional close with the Oedipal phase (see *Oedipus complex*), in which the relational triangle of father-mother-child takes on its specific form and is followed by the so-called period of latency serving the development of the ego. This then merges into a genital phase with the onset of puberty in which the partial drives are subordinated to the seeking of genital pleasure characteristic of mature sexuality.

## Ego psychology

Although ego psychology was already mentioned by Freud in earlier writings it was in 1923 with "The Ego and the Id" that he laid the foundations for psychoanalytic ego psychology in which he developed the structural model with the three *agencies* ego, id and superego. In this paradigm, ego is an integrating agency working to mediate between the demands of the id, the superego, and external reality and trying, where there are divergences between them, to find a balance or a way out.

The id contains the drive and more physical needs while the superego censors and judges as the praising and prohibiting agency representing values, norms, and ideals. All three agencies are located partly in the *unconscious* and partly in consciousness.

The ego with its ego functions (e.g., perception, thinking, deciding, and *defence*) is the central agency of action. It can fulfil its functions because a "displaceable energy" (Freud, 1923b, p. 43) is available which stems from desexualised and sublimated drive energy drawn away from *objects*. An important task of the ego is *defence*, which is set up against unpleasant, painful, threatening, and tabooed inner impulses. The *defence* mechanisms available for this depend on the particular ego structure (A. Freud, 1936) and contribute in pathological cases to the formation of symptoms.

Hartmann (1958) added to ideas about the tasks of *defence* mechanisms with the observation that they served adaption to external reality. For there to be normal psychical development and functioning he saw the necessity for particular ego functions to develop and be used free from conflict and for this he posited a *conflict-free ego-sphere*.

The psychic energy at the disposal of the ego he named *neutralised drive energy* which he saw as stemming from the two primary drives of aggression and sexuality as he called them (Hartmann, 1948). Hartmann (1950) also introduced the word *self* into psychoanalysis as a technical term. He used this term to refer to a person's own being which Freud had called *ich*—which had led to a difficulty (in German) in differentiating this from the *ich* (in Strachey's translation the ego) as agency in the framework of the structural theory. The inner images of self and object, to which all psychic processes finally relate, are called self-representation and object representation in Hartmann's terminology.

## Object relations psychology

While Freud emphasised the importance of the *object* he always saw it in connection with the drive and its gratification. By contrast, in the various object relation theories the importance of the early experiences of relationship with a significant *object* are given special emphasis. It is from the child-object interaction that the child develops his motivations, fears, modes of *defence*, and expectations for later relationships in his life. Melanie Klein was the first to focus on the early object relationship. For her the object relationship is essentially one imagined by the child, an internalised object relationship formed from the child's projections and introjections (Klein, 1932, 1946). The real *object* and the real object relationship may be quite different.

There is a contrast here with other object relation theories where the real experiences of relationship between child and object are more emphasised. In the "British object relations theory", whose most important representatives were Fairbairn, Guntrip, Sutherland, and Winnicott, an innate need for relation and bonding in an object relationship is assumed. Winnicott (1953) developed a model for the detachment from the primary object in what has become a famous concept: the *transitional object*.

In these theories, the decisive influence on the shaping of relationships in later life is attributed to the real, early experiences of relationship. For techniques in treatment these approaches lead to a far greater consideration of what happens in the relationship during therapy. *Transference* and *countertransference* serve significantly to draw inferences from early childhood experiences in relationships and to use these insights for the treatment.

## Self psychology

Self psychology developed as a logical counterpart to *object relations* psychology if we assume that the *libido* essentially *cathects* both the self and *objects*. The self is not a psychic agency but the psychic representation of images which a person has of himself. The founder of the self psychology school in psychoanalysis is Heinz Kohut (1971) who concerned himself with the treatment of patients with narcissistic disorders and with the question of maintaining narcissistic homeostasis. He observed in narcissistically disturbed patients the need to have another person act as echo and offer confirmation, praise, or even admiration. In the treatment, according to Kohut, the analyst becomes this person: a particular *transference* emerges in which the analyst is turned into such an *object* that mirrors positive feelings. Kohut calls this *transference* the mirror *transference*. Kohut also observed in these patients a tendency to idealise the analyst—to take him for omniscient, omnipotent, and perfect.

Kohut started from the position that primary narcissism—the existence of which he assumes, following Freud—experiences natural disturbances through the limitations to which maternal care is necessarily subjected. In order to compensate for and regulate the disturbed narcissistic balance, the child, as he saw it, develops two archaic structures, the grandiose self and a self-object of the idealised parent imago. With them the child experiences himself as omnipotent.

In normal, relatively undisturbed development, through constant confrontations with reality, the grandiose self and the idealised parent imago are continuously reworked, corrected and increasingly drawn into the self, above all in the formation of a superego. In a disturbed development, feelings of being too small, dependent, unworthy, and incapable are warded off with the activation of the grandiose self which opposes the feeling of being nothing with a feeling of omnipotence and grandiosity.

## Intersubjective and relational theories

From about the 1980s onward various psychoanalytic theories have been developed which emphasise a person's relatedness to the other or others. Though there were representatives of an interpersonal psychoanalysis in the 40s and 50s—of whom Sullivan, Fromm, Horney, and Fromm-Reichmann are the best known—the main schools of thought in psychoanalysis such as ego psychology, self psychology, and the Kleinian school were decided advocates of the analysis of the inner world.

The swing which Altmeyer and Thomä (2006) call the "intersubjective turn in psychoanalysis" may well, above all, have been the discoveries of modern research into infant development (pp. 13 ff.) which proved the intersubjective development of psychic structures and functions (Dornes, 2006). This changed perspective was supported by a social-philosophical school of thought which sees self-conscious human existence as essentially grounded in the perception of the other and orientation to the other (see, e.g., Honneth, 1992). This line of thought has also been taken up by the intersubjective approach in psychoanalysis.

The common ground between the various approaches of an intersubjective and relational psychoanalysis, whose most prominent representative was Stephen Mitchell, is the assumption that the human psyche is formed in the relationships of earliest childhood and intersubjective processes of a person, that these relational experiences are re-created in later interpersonal relationships, that in the course of a treatment a psychoanalyst is also woven into the matrix, and that in a treatment it is a question of working on a common understanding of the patient's history and of the exchange between analyst and patient in the treatment situation. It is not only a question of reconstructing a historical truth—something that can never succeed—but rather of developing an intersubjective narrative truth (Spence, 1982). As Hoffman (1998) argues in more detail in a social-constructivist approach, the results of psychoanalytic treatment and newly gained insights into it are thus to be regarded as a construction creating sense and meaning.

## The concept of mentalisation and the development of thoughts

The capacity for mentalisation is viewed today as one of the indispensable, central psychic functions without which psychic health cannot be achieved. Mentalisation means the connection of basic psychic processes such as drive impulses, primary phantasies, or unfiltered affects with psychological and contextual meanings as they are produced in a subtle exchange process between mother and child in the first year of life (Fonagy, Gergely, Jurist & Target, 2002; Dornes, 2006). This means near-to-body psychic events such as the primary affects (joy, anger, fear, disgust, sadness, curiosity, contempt) are linked with a moment and a context and thus receive a psychological meaning. They are no longer experienced, as by a newborn infant, as an incomprehensible storm of excitation of pleasant or unpleasant quality. Such a connection is built up in a subtle, reciprocal exchange between mother and child which Fonagy, Gergely, Jurist, and Target (2002) conceptualise as the "social biofeedback model of maternal mirroring". A new level of understanding, attribution, and reflection on the infant's own states is formed.

In this interaction, the mother takes in the infant's affect through identifying with it. In this way she not only observes but also experiences the infant's inner state. She reacts, however, to this state with her own experience of life and composure, and therefore differently from the way the infant reacts. This difference is mirrored back to the child. In doing this she modulates the infant's affects through *marking*, which means the pronounced, mirroring back of an affect of the same category, changed to some extent and not just identical.

For instance, she takes in the infant's anger but does not mirror back the state of "being beside herself" she might have in a real state of anger, but rather a state of mild annoyance. In this way she takes the sting out of the infant's violent, perhaps overwhelming affect of anger. She conveys to the child that one may well be annoyed that the milk is not as yet flowing into the breast but that one doesn't have to be beside oneself because of that. What is conveyed to the infant here is that his anger is caused by the milk not arriving, that there is a context and also that his anger is out of proportion: a much milder form is enough. At the same time the mother calms the infant through her softened affect-mirroring which, however, does not deny the infant's anger and its justification. The infant, for its part, can identify with this. In the interaction the infant's anger receives a confirmation, softening, and contextualisation, and through this he takes in a meaning as a signal for a self state and as a means of communication for the future.

This form of mirroring back leads to a "referential decoupling" between the affective return on the mother's part and the infant's original affective state. As a result the infant's anger and the mother's response do not clash spontaneously and impulsively because the mother does not simply throw the ball back: she takes it up, turns it into a soft ball, giving it back carefully a little later. Her response is decoupled from the infant's anger. Marking and referential decoupling enable the infant to differentiate between his own and the mother's mirrored affect—the beginning of thinking. At the same time the first foundations of the ability to symbolise is laid, namely being able to express something with the affect, which allows a self-reflective distancing from the immediate affective experience. The differentiation between "marked" and realistic expression, for instance between the mother's playful, pretended annoyance and her real anger in another situation, establishes a generalised communication code, a symbol system.

The mother shows "I can be angry" and I can "act" being angry. The "acting" of anger is its symbolisation, its imaginary production in the absence of real anger, just as the word "horse" evokes the image of a horse but does not bring a real horse on stage. This kind of interaction establishes the principle of symbolisation. Modulating affect-mirroring plays a role not only in affect integration and the development of thinking, which is founded on symbolisation, but also in the existential self-confirmation of the infant.

It conveys to the baby "the experience of causal efficacy" when he experiences himself as the active originator of an emotional state in the mother. The baby experiences himself as someone who can have an effect, for instance, evoke a certain response in the mother. This is an experience of being alive, an experience of power and influence.

Built on the foundation of observations in developmental psychology, this theory of the production of the meaning of psychic and interpersonal processes that is also of a differential cognition and therefore of thinking, had already been formulated in different language by Bion (1962b). He developed his container/contained model for the processes of exchange between mother and child from clinical observations. In this model mother and child form one processing unit for certain psychic processes and states. The child conveys psychic elements that he has not understood or cannot understand to the mother as the container. She processes or digests these contents or elements, "the contained", to give a structure to the information which the child can take in with the help of her transformative capability, the alpha function. She gives the transformed information back as $\alpha$-elements. This model of an intersubjective process between mother and child is also a model for psychoanalytic treatment.

## On the psychology of puberty and adolescence

Puberty and adolescence, with growth in size and strength and the onset of sexual maturity, not only bring major changes to the body, they are also periods of psychological turmoil (Blos, 1973; Bohleber, 1999; Gunter, 2006a, 2008; Laufer & Laufer, 1989; Streeck-Fischer, 1994, 2004). The adolescent's body schema or body self-representation changes because the adolescent's own body is experienced differently. Since the sense of identity is essentially physically determined it is shaken by these changes. Sexual maturity with the sexual desires and actions it brings on often leads to feelings of guilt and shame and fears of punishment.

The mental-emotional system of *defence* is overtaxed with these new libidinal needs so that temporarily the adolescent shows a tendency to impulsive and regressive behaviour. Oedipal conflicts are revived. They find expression in bouts of rivalry between father and son, mother and daughter, or in the sharp and emphatic dissociation from the opposite-sex parent as a sign of *defence* against incestuous desires. The parents begin to be less cathected with libido. Because often no love *object* outside the family is as yet available what develops is an increasing narcissistic cathexis of the self. This manifests for example in an exaggeration of self (Blos, 1973) taking on an appearance which is always culturally and often sub-culturally determined.

Independently of whether the adolescent has a heterosexual or homosexual orientation, part of the narcissistic libido is directed towards a homosexual object choice. Particularly in early adolescence this grouping can often serve to ward off and channel sexual fears better. The forming of same-age same-sex groups is widespread among boys and girls. In these groups the homosexual choice of object provides an important sense of solidarity. The partial withdrawal of libidinal cathexis from the parents introduces a further detachment from them which is necessary for the integration of the young person into society.

Feelings over the loss of the loved objects are connected with phases of sad-to-tragic moods. In place of these first objects the young increasingly turn with their libido to activities in the intellectual, scientific, cultural, and moral fields.

The increased narcissistic cathexis of the self carries with it the danger that differentiation between self and object is weakened and objects may take on the quality of self-objects, as they did in the early narcissistic phase of infancy when the infant could not yet recognise objects as being independent but rather regarded them as its living tools, there to obey its wishes—that is, its self-objects. This, in turn, means that the testing of reality is endangered, which is one source of adolescent daydreaming—inner reality gains in importance over external reality and at the same time there is a strong tendency to translate inner states into action.

These complicated inner processes are hard for adolescents to understand and they make puberty and adolescence a period of conflicts with the adult world full of *transference* figures with whom adolescents need to "wrestle". At the same time, however, they need to mark a boundary between these adults and themselves.

## CHAPTER FOUR

# Areas in which psychoanalytic social work is applied

As explained in the preceding chapters, psychoanalytic social work has to do with a specific way of reflecting on social work and on the relations which are part of the process of this work. It is concerned with how actions in the real world, more or less competent social actions, affect and are affected by processes of inner experience (cf. Chapter 8).

Thus psychoanalytic social work is not simply a further, specific form of assistance in the education or integration of a client, in accordance with the Children's Act 1989 but is characterised by a special form of reflection on the dynamics of the relations between helper and client which enable an individual accommodation of the forms of assistance offered to the specific needs of the person entitled to this help.

As such it can be applied in educational counselling, in social group work, in educational support, in socio-pedagogical family aid, in education in day care groups, in children's homes and support settings, in forms of supported housing, in intensive socio-pedagogical individual counselling, and further areas.

Although in principle psychoanalytic social work can be used across the full range of assistance measures, some typical areas of application and forms of psychoanalytic social work will be briefly presented in the following material as they have evolved and proved their worth in practice.

This more general characterisation of currently established areas of the practice of psychoanalytic social work is enlarged on in Chapters Six to Twelve with detailed accounts of specific problem areas. Chapter Fifteen depicts examples of the practice of psychoanalytic social work, detailing the range of diverse, complementary forms of assistance offered. In the present chapter part one provides an overview of the most important problem areas in children, adolescents, and adults and part two introduces forms of psychoanalytic social work.

## 1. Areas in which psychoanalytic social work is applied

### Psychotic and autistic children and adolescents

One of the classic fields of psychoanalytic social work is the care, treatment, and social integration of autistic and psychotic children and adolescents (cf. Becker 1991; Becker & Nedelmann, 1987; Bettelheim, 1950, 1967; Verein für Psychoanalytische Sozialarbeit, 1993, 2000). In the case of most of these children and adolescents social and school or workplace integration is considerably impaired. According to the extent of psychosocial impairment, intensive assistance is required for social integration and permanent stabilisation. This is particularly so in cases of aggressive conduct disorders, social withdrawal and refusal to interact, imminent or repeated psychotic breakdowns, signs of a developing state of neglect, or overtaxing of family structures.

Inpatient treatment in a clinic for child and adolescent psychiatry can certainly be helpful but by virtue of its short-term character this is no substitute for intensive, long-term psychosocial forms of support. Psychiatric and psychotherapeutic treatment in day clinics is in general also insufficient to help the patient and family to achieve long-term stability. Often schools and workshops for disabled people are in need of counselling when they are confronted with the behaviour of these children and young people which is in many cases hard to understand and frightening, or even bizarre.

Whereas children with infant or early autism and mental disabilities are indeed accepted by classic institutions for the disabled, the care and social integration of psychotic children and adolescents, and also of those with pronounced Asperger's syndrome and disorders in social behaviour, often proves decidedly difficult. They fall, so to speak, through the cracks between psychiatric and socio-pedagogical services. To care for and assist them requires sufficient psychiatric knowledge and also an appreciation of the inner dynamics and the resulting crises in relationships which threaten to break the mould of care. Settings for the care of these children often comprise outpatient forms of help involving the family and school, integration in the workplace, and also admission to specialised group homes. The aim here is to stabilise them at least to the point where they can find a place to live in the regular institutions for the care of the disabled or the mentally ill.

*Personality disorders and disorders in the development of personality*

Personality disorders are characterised by deeply rooted, inappropriate patterns of behaviour in a range of situations restricting a person's ability to perform at work and in social life. They begin in childhood or youth and lead to impairments in various areas of functioning and in relationships to others. Even though the diagnosis of a personality disorder in childhood and adolescence is disputed, severe impairments of this kind not infrequently also occur in children and adolescents. As a rule they require both age-appropriate psychiatric treatment, comprehensive measures for integration in school, workplace, and the social sphere and also support for a mental and emotional development as close as possible to normal. Above all adolescents with the most common serious psychiatric diagnosis of this age group, namely that of an emotionally unstable personality structure of the borderline type, pose considerable problems for the children's and young people's institutions which have care of them. Problems arise out of the instability of these young persons' relationships, the often rapid swings from idealisation to devaluation, their unrestrained *acting out* in external reality of feelings of anger, depression, and emptiness, and their tendency to trigger conflicts in a team or between the various institutions involved. An understanding of the reasons for aggressive and even threatening behaviour can make an appropriate and clear reaction possible. This may, in one case, be the clear setting of boundaries involving a psychiatric clinic or the police, in another case it may be the attempt to de-escalate by offering a space in the relationship to the social worker for the deep, warded-off anxieties. In addition these adolescents often shift their unbearable feelings onto other people, particularly those who concern themselves more closely with them. This could for instance be the social worker. Affective entanglements can arise through these *unconscious transferences* and can often defy disentanglement (see *projective identification* in the Glossary).

All this demands systematic reflection on the dynamics of the client's inner world, the dynamics of his relationships, and of *transference* in order to gain an appropriate relation to him between closeness and distance. It has often been observed that, if such dynamics are not sufficiently thought over, an initially major effort for the client when paired with marked affectionate attention is followed by bitter disappointment when, in the process of work, the destructive and negative sides of the client gradually gain the upper hand, frequently precisely at the moment when he begins to develop a sense of trust.

Psychoanalytic social work serves here to develop a picture of the inner world of the client, one which helps to integrate the various aspects of his psyche and maintain the social worker's own ability to think and reflect. It is what enables the social worker in the frequently violent, sometimes insulting conflicts in the team or between institutions, such as local authority children's and young people's services, hospitals, and non-government agencies for young people, to understand these as the staging of a desperate inner defensive struggle and to defuse the conflict through understanding. It is also helpful in reducing the mental and emotional strains on the carer which result from the intensity of the working relationship.

Settings involving a number of staff are often required in the work with such adolescents to enable the client's positive and negative *transference* to be distributed over several people. *Splittings* of this kind are often only perceptible in supervision. For a certain time they can, however, be the precondition for maintaining any kind of supportive or therapeutic relationship (Bruns, 1995). Flexible and constantly re-reflected accommodation of the concrete framework conditions to the psychic structure and dynamics of the client is therefore essential in order to limit his or her destructive *acting out* and tendencies to break off contact. For these adolescents, too, a wide spectrum of measures needs to be available—ranging from day clinic programmes through supported housing and integration in the workplace to full inpatient treatment, whereby the more intensive the form of care offered the more the balance between closeness and distance requires constant and intensive reflection.

## Antisocial developments

A further area of psychoanalytic social work is that of antisocial developments which particularly affect adolescence. On the whole, clients with this condition are not amenable to a psychotherapeutic treatment although the roots of the state are rather clear—frequently chronic deprivation or experience of violence in the family. The antisocial *defence* structure is often absolutely cemented because allowing access to his needy, softer sides is experienced by the client as too threatening and painful. For this reason more can be achieved with sound teaching work. Classics in this field and still well worth reading, although not up-to-date as regards theoretical background, are August Aichhorn's *Wayward Youth* (1925) and Siegfried Bernfeld's *Sisyphus or the Limits of Education* (1925).

From the viewpoint of psychoanalysis the essential thing with children and adolescents showing antisocial tendencies or marked antisocial developments is to create a framework in which these young people can experience enough security in a place where they have something to hold onto. This applies in both senses, namely holding structures in the sense of firm boundaries and holding in the sense of being held and accepted even with their unbearable feelings of anger, abandonment, and humiliation.

Winnicott's (1984) concept of the antisocial tendency is very helpful in this context. He emphasises that the antisocial tendency develops because of a failure of the child's environment. Antisocial behaviour forces the environment to take up a position and is therefore to be read as a child's appeal for someone to take control while showing tolerance and understanding. An understanding of the inner dynamics of an antisocial child or adolescent, which are staged in the form of offences in the external world, allows room for an appropriate way of dealing with them.

Two extremes are to be avoided: the one is looking the other way—often observed in residential groups which may be too challenged by this behaviour—and the other is providing a rigid system of rules without any building of relationship to the young person. Particularly for these adolescents, who have been so disappointed by their environment, relationships are essential and are taxed to the utmost. Psychoanalytic social work, with its effort to understand, helps to see the hidden neediness and thus take the adolescent's side in an appropriate way. One could say it in Winnicott's words, "The work is only worth doing if it is personal and if those who are doing the work are not overburdened" (1984, p. 185).

The aggressive dynamics are frequently fed by the client's highly negative and devaluing self images which, in contrast to the common perception, do not stem from a lack of conscience but on the contrary from a conscience which is particularly severe and persecutory. Adolescents often report that the act of committing the offence represents a kind of breaking out of their imprisonment in self-devaluation and feelings of guilt. The moment of narcissistic triumph associated with it does not, however, last long and the cycle begins again. In addition the act creates a concrete reason for existing feelings of guilt and worthlessness which seem in this way to become more bearable for a time. To change these dynamics, first of all the feeling of being worthless has to be overcome, as is for example attempted in experiential education projects. Further, the enjoyment that the young person has drawn from narcissistic triumph needs to be replaced by other means of self-affirmation.

The psychoanalytic approach enables social workers to keep these dynamics in view and work on them in the everyday relationship. The setting can range from outreach services through experiential education approaches to full inpatient admissions. In certain cases therapeutic work in the strict sense of the word can gradually be built up through normal everyday encounters.

## Work with severely developmentally impaired, disabled, and chronically ill children

Disabled, severely developmentally impaired, and chronically ill children carry an additional risk of developing psychological disorders. Their families, too, are under strain in many forms. Even if the majority of families affected are able to cope with these burdens, in individual cases intensive educational support may be required to accompany the therapeutic and medical treatment for the child. In these cases psychoanalytic social work above all works towards understanding dysfunctional coping strategies and their function as *defence* systems with the aim of developing and using the often hidden resources there. Serious barriers to the child's development can develop from the family's feelings of guilt and shame, their fears of how the illness will develop, and their strict suppression of aggressive feelings towards the child, which are necessary for its development. Moreover, there are their fears of failure, of being constricted by the illness or disability, and of its becoming the focal point for the whole family. If no improvement is achieved through the usual interventions, such as psycho-education, comprehensive information for family and child with chronic illnesses, linking to self-help groups, activating support, assisted family holidays, then increasing such assistance is generally of no use. It is then necessary to investigate and change the dynamics which have developed in the family and social relations around the sick child.

At this point psychoanalytic social work is focussed on the counselling and support of the parents and also counselling for the school. This is usually supplemented by educational and therapeutic work with the child itself which can be supported and extended by forms of treatment of a more functional nature such as physiotherapy. The work is aimed at the prevention of secondary damage and forms of developmental impairment. It can help avoid the need for the child to be taken out of his family and placed in an institution for the disabled.

## Mental and emotional disorders in parents

The strain and burden on the children of parents with mental and emotional disorders—frequently alcohol or drug dependency—have increasingly become a focus of professional concern and discussion. They play a large part in young people's support measures. The parents often try to evade any form of influence exerted by public authorities. This not infrequently leads to escalations between those offering help and the family concerned so that there is always a danger that contact will be broken off. This danger can be countered by ensuring that work with the children is accompanied by a form of contact with the parents which has been thought through in therapeutic terms, which avoids the giving of advice, relying in its place on the building of relationship and alliance with the parents too. Only when their needy side and encoded search for help is recognised and skilfully answered is there any chance of winning them over to cooperation in the assistance offered to the children and to themselves.

In such scenarios psychoanalytic social work aims at arranging for parents and children to receive support from different people. Each member of the family is to be given a space for himself and his mental and emotional needs. Bringing the different aspects together can take place in regular parental sessions to include the person working with the children, or in complete family sessions. In these dispositions the psychoanalytic social worker will find herself in a field of perceptible tension. On the one hand she has to perceive and take up the needs both of parents and children, which also means dealing with them in confidentiality and responsibility, but, on the other hand, she has a specific position as guarantor of the well-being of the children.

In cases where the best interests of children seem considerably endangered and this danger cannot be averted by the intervention carried out, this guarantor position will lead the social worker to inform the authorities and suggest taking a child into care as a last resort according to the Children's Act 1989.

The possibilities offered by psychoanalytic reflection in social work enable those involved to achieve a more rational weighing of such radical measures. In this way two dangers can be avoided: action for action's sake, and an ignoring of the child's endangerment on the grounds that in a particular case there is "only" psychological impairment and that physical abuse plays no role.

Psychoanalytic social work can also pursue the goal of winning the parents' cooperation via an understanding of their own neediness. This enables them to identify with the needs of their child and give up their resistance to having him placed away from home.

## Disorganised adults with mental disorders

In practice, so far, psychoanalytic social work has most often been restricted to children, adolescents, young adults, and their families. There are, however, also reports of experience with working with severely socially deprived and emotionally disturbed adults, for instance adults with severe personality disorders, chronic addiction illnesses, or the socially marginalised. Here, working with the concepts of social work and socio-psychiatry, one will first make sure that living conditions are improved. In the course of instrumental help given (help dealing with authorities, management of finances, etc.) a personal relationship between social worker and client is built up and this is affected by all the turbulence, described above, which marks the life of these people.

The goal will often be limited and will confine itself to making life more bearable and stable without aiming at a fundamental healing and complete social integration. Nevertheless, building on the strengths of its methods, psychoanalytic social work can tackle the way clients have neglected their own needs, the way they have turned their hardened disappointment and anger against themselves, and can address the instability of relationships. Work in these areas can set developments in motion.

The setting is in most cases likely to be one-to-one and will take practical real life problems into consideration with the differing approaches of socio-psychiatry and psychoanalytic social work complementing each other. In practical terms such help can be embedded in socio-psychiatric aid, in care, in management of finances for adults, or in outreach services.

## 2. Settings for psychoanalytic social work

In the following section the most important forms of psychoanalytic social work—their settings—are described. Most of these settings were already mentioned above in the section on areas of indication. Here only their essential structure and a few important aspects will be briefly touched on. Psychoanalytic social work has up to now had its main base in young people's services which is why these fields of work dominate in the following description. Separate chapters (Chapters Six and Seven) have been devoted to mediation with its rather different structure and to psychoanalytic social work in early education and early intervention.

### Non-residential measures

Non-residential measures in psychoanalytic social work are frequently to be found in the borderland between child psychotherapy and socio-pedagogic intervention. Typically, indication for it is given when children show signs of neglect or where there are clear signs that the parents are overtaxed and where these are accompanied by mental-emotional problems of the children or the parents, when relationship conflicts cannot be sufficiently diffused through educational interventions, and when in cases of disability further factors such as retarded development or chronic illnesses appear which require therapeutic alongside educational measures.

Frequently, families in need of help cannot be relied on to get a child to outpatient appointments regularly. In addition, the parents are without any clear idea of how to bring up the children or run things in the home, so that accompanying parental counselling, as is often offered in outpatient psychotherapy, is not sufficient. The families have to be visited in their own surroundings and to be counselled there. This is often the only way to ensure parental cooperation. Sometimes a family "help" with socio-pedagogical background is needed. Providing an intensive and thought-out relationship can, however, reduce the need for such practical care, since in this way the inner need structures and resources of the family are perceived and taken into consideration. One could say the family's neediness is indirectly satisfied in such a relationship and not via instrumental assistance.

In outpatient measures of this kind, as opposed to outpatient psychotherapy, it is relatively easy to arrange for a multi-person setting. For instance, one or more members of staff can work with one or more children while others are responsible for the parents.

The aim of outpatient care for adolescents and young adults is, first of all, to get their real life circumstances into some sort of order. They simply cannot cope with practical tasks such as the ordering of their finances and living conditions, training, applications for jobs, and the like. Their families frequently offer no support and so necessary steps are not taken and the young people find themselves helpless in a growing labyrinth of problems. Psychoanalytic social workers not only accompany their clients to a potential employer or landlord but also work with them to understand the mental and emotional processes that keep leading to failure.

Provocative behaviour to a landlord may have its roots in the client's seeing the mould on his ceiling as a sign of intentional disregard for his needs. One adolescent with this notion in his mind flew into such a rage that he attacked the landlord and so provoked being given notice. In another case a young person had such paranoid fears that he could not bring himself to flush his urine down the toilet but kept it in bottles in his room and later poured it out in the garden. Fears of this kind can only be overcome without painful social consequences if they are understood in a supportive framework and can be recognised as the subjective expression of unresolved mental and emotional conflicts.

At any rate the various elements of outpatient care in the framework of psychoanalytic social work not only have to be aligned to one another but also reflected on in the team. For this reason supervision of the measures taken and a bringing together of the various aspects of *transference* are particularly important in such contexts.

## Residential homes and groups

In purely formal terms the group homes which are based on the principles of psychoanalytic social work do not differ greatly from other residential centres run by government and other organisations. They will, however, usually take in more children and adolescents who show considerable mental and emotional problems, mostly with severe psychiatric symptoms.

We have established a residential home of this kind for autistic and psychotic children as well as a community for autistic and psychotic adolescents and young people, usually suffering from schizophrenia. Even after longer spells of hospital treatment it was not possible to integrate them in schools and/or work or even generally available support systems. The home was set up nearly twenty years ago when it proved impossible to find a placement for an autistic patient with marked psychotic symptoms after a series of hospital stays, either in a local authority supported housing scheme or in an institution for the disabled. After living in the home for five years he was sufficiently stabilised to be able to live in a flat of his own, linked to a home for those with mental health issues, and for the last fifteen years has been working in a workshop for the disabled.

The difference between this home and the usual kind for adolescents is that here the team meet regularly to think through the *transference* and *countertransference* dynamics. Also, the staff can set up relationships tailored to the individual and can integrate them into an overall concept instead of offering the range of educational and other interventions in modular form. Reflecting with the client on the dynamics of conflicts and the range of his or her relationships enables staff to perceive interactions consciously even in everyday situations and to react to young clients appropriately.

In this way social work is underpinned by an understanding of mental-emotional problems. It is not changed into some kind of psychotherapy in day-to-day life. Attention is paid to avoiding setting up any imbalance of power through the use of clever interpretations. Quite the contrary, psychological knowledge is used here purely as background knowledge in dealing with the client's day-to-day life, a process which may well also include the use of an instructional setting of boundaries, while catering for the inner needs of the client. Alongside having regular supervision, at least some members of staff should have sufficient experience in working with people with severe mental and emotional disorders and if possible should have worked for a longer period of time in a psychiatric clinic. In addition, depending on the age of the young residents, cooperation is needed with a child and adolescent psychiatrist or psychiatrist for adults, and also with a clinic willing to admit residents for a crisis intervention. The supportive framework needed for the residents must also be set up for the institutions so that work can be assured of a solid foundation.

An important factor in psychoanalytic social work in a residential setting is the consideration of the inner meaning for the client of contact with reality outside the group home. For instance, leaving the home to get to school or work can trigger separation anxieties so that it may be necessary, at least for a time, for a resident to be accompanied. Clients may also experience everyday work as threatening to the narcissistic delusions of grandeur they cannot do without. Thus any kind of job will be rejected in a grandiose gesture as being beneath their dignity. If it also takes these *defence* processes into consideration, social work carried out in a spirit of patience is in a position to set gradual changes in motion. Finally, the relation between group dynamics and individual psychodynamics requires reflection since group processes offer the possibility of externalising unbearable mental-emotional conflicts via projections into external reality.

## Supported housing

Normally, forms of supported housing are designed for young people who need far less help than is offered in a group home. But there are often adolescents who need relatively intensive support, in particular those with emotionally unstable personality disorders of the borderline type or those whose development shows antisocial traits. Some of them are, however, almost impossible to integrate into a group since they use group situations to avoid the seemingly unbearable and frightening confrontation with themselves. These adolescents destroy groups, totally disregard rules and become threatening out of a fear of committed relationships that seem to them too constricting. The result is that some of them have more than once had to leave such programmes. A less regulated supported living model can be an alternative in such cases. Admittedly, however, this involves the danger of their descending into neglect or producing unmanageable problems over their massive *acting out* in this setting, too.

In these sometimes desperate cases psychoanalytic social work can offer the framework in which to keep up the constant re-regulating of relations needed to achieve a kind of appropriate, medium distance. Through allotting the various responsibilities to different members of staff, as already mentioned, the dynamics of *defence* can be responded to and a tolerable setting can be developed to deal with them. Help is directed first of all to the practical necessities of life such as maintenance, accommodation, work, job applications, etc. This work, which is carried out together with the client, introduces a "third" in the relationship and can mitigate the adolescent's marked fears both of entering into and also of losing relationships.

Psychoanalytic social work thus always sees practical support in dealing with everyday life as an opportunity to build relationships that can carry a certain load. In other respects what has been said in relation to non-residential measures applies here too.

## Integration into school and work

Compulsory school attendance, and with it the educational task of schools, also comprises provision for children with marked mental-emotional and behavioural disorders. Frequently schools, including special schools, are stretched to their limits and find themselves sucked into dynamics of relationships and *transference* they cannot cope with using only the means at their disposal.

In the case of mentally and emotionally impaired older adolescents it is still often possible to set up moderately satisfactory schooling. However, as soon as schooling is completed and the transition to the world of work approaches in many cases it becomes clear that the requirements of the world of work are beyond the scope of what these adolescents can handle. The programmes for integration set up by job centres and measures for rehabilitation are mainly tailored to other target groups. Sheltered workshops for mentally disabled people or workshops for those with mental and emotional disorders are often unable to cope with these adolescents.

For young people with such mental and emotional symptoms psychoanalytic social work can often achieve the decisive helpful step towards integration. The aid may consist of direct work with them in the sense of educational, therapeutic work and can include offers of help to the family but it can also, at least for certain periods, take the form of the psychoanalytic social worker accompanying the adolescent to school, to work, or to the vocational training centre. This can achieve a wide range of things: for example, a child or adolescent may only be able to "bear" herself in a group or work situation if another person, acting as a *container*, takes in something of her mental-emotional state and thus relieves her of a part of the strain. Psychological and interpersonal conflicts can be "caught" and made understandable with the help of a psychoanalytic social worker so that with this accompaniment the client develops socially appropriate ways of behaving. The inducing of violent *countertransference* reactions by staff often caused by difficult adolescent behaviour can be reduced and this brings about a better working atmosphere.

School and work requirements often have to be aligned to the impairments and over-sensitivities of the children and adolescents in question. At times schedules, dealing with getting to and from school or work, coping with tasks and similar things, need to be adjusted to particular inner problems of the young person. Social contacts outside the actual functional work tasks present many of these children and adolescents with a particular challenge because they feel so awkward in them. And finally, schools and institutions concerned with integration into work are often glad of counselling over this particular clientele.

## Counselling institutions

One indirect form of psychoanalytic social work is the counselling of institutions concerned with difficult psychosocial problem areas. Among these are institutions for youth welfare as well as schools, programmes for getting difficult youngsters into work, child protective services, and other social institutions. The commonest form of institutional counselling is the use of supervision sessions attended by staff members of the institution who do not work on the basis of psychoanalytic social work. But youth protection services, too, use support from psychoanalytic social work in carrying out a "clearing" or social pedagogic diagnosis.

## Social counselling, debt regulation, management of finances, and similar

In the classic social counselling settings, too, psychoanalytic social work can be an effective approach. Marginalised and socially decompensating clients often show little tendency to go to counselling in the widest sense but they use the services offered here often with the hidden aim of finding a human relationship. In this way public authority financial counselling of clients who have lost all social contacts can be used to regard an officially imposed management of a client's finances not only as an instrument to stabilise external living conditions but also as a chance to gain access to his or her inner world. It is a fact that clients often tell such staff about all their conflicts, mental and emotional problems, and breakdowns. An understanding of the mental-emotional dynamics at work here protects carers from having illusions of being able to heal this person but also enables them to stay in a relationship to the client and not sink into a resigned lack of interest.

In the course of counselling work carers can experience hope, disappointment, anger, and resignation; they feel of no value, see their work as pointless, and suffer from feelings of shame and guilt. These feelings are the expression of their *countertransference*. When they understand this they can enter into stable counselling relationships, reduce the danger of the client's breaking off relations and also their own resignation.

## CHAPTER FIVE

# Psychoanalytic social work in the wider context of social and therapeutic assistance: points of contact and differences

Psychoanalytic social work defines itself primarily in terms of its practice as a form of social work and so it employs the full range of forms of intervention and setting possibilities which have been developed in social work, are based on its theory and practice, and are regarded as helpful. Among these are low needs outpatient support on a case-by-case basis, for instance focussing on expanding social competence and the ability to build relationships constructively, and the support offered in claiming and using available institutional aid. The range covers family-orientated help in its various forms as well as semi-inpatient and fully inpatient measures.

In psychoanalytically orientated social work a central focus in offering these forms of help is on creating more favourable conditions for the clients to develop in, while at the same time keeping the aspect of the relationship with them constantly in view. This applies to the clients' relationships within their families and the dynamics prevailing there and also to relationships in their social environment. All these relationships are investigated and seen with reference to their emotional importance for those involved and with reference to how they may block a client's development. This work in and on relationships between clients and social workers is what psychoanalytic social workers perceive as the heart of their task.

Correspondingly, in its theoretical orientation the focus of its work is on constant reflection on *unconscious* relationships, structures, and processes, which we can best grasp in the concept of the *object relation,* to use the technical term. Psychoanalytic social work is prepared for an inner state in the *subject* (here the client) in which there is a will to independence, a cleaving to what is his own way, and therefore resistance to "well-meaning" social interventions. Linked to these there may well be a narrowing of thought, fixations, blinkered outlook, and considerable impairments in the ability to take part in social life, in other words the client suffers from "being the person he is".

Theory and practice of classic social work action and of social pedagogic concepts of development are supplemented in psychoanalytic social work with an active focus on the specific mental and emotional structures of the individual and on the interactional processes in the family and social environment that stem from these structures. For the action taken in social work this differentiation means that no solid body of intervention techniques can be created for psychoanalytic social work and that it does not represent any further specific technique. Instead it sees itself as the application of what we have outlined here, namely the inclusion of inner processes in individuals and groups as a factor in all areas of social work. In this sense it extends the many intervention techniques and methods already developed in the social field by introducing a changed understanding of them. On the other hand this perspective brings it into a certain proximity to forms of therapeutic intervention.

As to content, the boundaries are fluid between psychoanalytic social work and therapeutic interventions in the stricter sense and in transitions from the one to the other. In terms of form, compared to therapy the area in which psychoanalytic social work exercises influence is far closer to the real life and environment of the client and more involved in it. To put it in slightly simplified terms, a basic precondition for psychoanalytic social work is created when the psychosocial difficulties and impairments are of such a nature that a therapy in the classic sense, with its relatively clear setting, seems impossible or has to be regarded as offering little or no promise of success.

In the following pages of this chapter we will be touching on some of the fields in which it may seem helpful to clarify points of contact with neighbouring approaches and areas of difference from them.

## Family therapy

The views and forms of intervention of systemic family therapy have gained widespread currency in social work in the form of adaptions. This is not the place to describe the whole range of systemic family therapy developments in social work. Despite all theoretical differences a systemic perspective and the viewpoint of psychoanalytic social work have this in common: that the embedding of the individual in his family and social system is seen as significant. In the view of both schools of thought many of the symptoms and problems affecting the families in question, with which the social worker is also therefore confronted, can only be sufficiently understood if the corresponding interdependencies are taken into consideration and incorporated into work with the client.

It would be a naive view which suggested that by simply taking a child out of the family of an alcoholic in decompensation one could expect his problems to be solved. A social worker working systemically would perhaps point out that the antisocial symptoms of the eleven-year-old involved had the function of stabilising the family and shaking the parents out of their preoccupation with alcohol, even maybe of bringing social institutions in on the scene. She would therefore possibly point to the considerable dangers both for the parents and for the child that such a destabilisation of the system would produce if the removal of the child from its home were imposed.

A social worker with a psychoanalytic social work approach would possibly also argue in a very similar way and would point to the *unconscious* identification of the boy with the destructive and autodestructive sides of the parents, as well as to the resulting powerful guilt feelings and psychological need for reparation. In any case the conflicts of loyalty and the bond between the boy and his parents would have to be taken into consideration in planning further help.

It would be a misunderstanding of the psychoanalytic perspective to assume, therefore, that in the course of such considerations only the possible traumatisations of early childhood would be seen as relevant.

Traumatisations are of interest in so far as they create, or have in the past created, mental and emotional structures and patterns of reaction and behaviour; these, however, only become relevant in connection with a current conflictual set of relationships. What are significant in the present are the relationship problems in the here and now of the family on the one hand and in the conflicts with the intervening social workers on the other—seen in psychoanalytic terms, the *transference*. These problems need to be understood and not dismissed as dusty past history. So much in brief for the essential points of similarity and contact between the two schools of thought.

From our perspective the differences emerge, above all, in two points:

1. Resources are orientated in a sometimes exaggerated and seemingly one-track way, running the danger of ignoring or even "whitewashing over" impairments, disadvantage, and lack of social participation and so ignoring the enormous suffering of clients. By contrast psychoanalytic social work holds on to a concept of the *subject*, who may well be susceptible to change but whose fundamental structures are persistent, full of contradictions, and determined by emotions and needs. Above all, emotions and needs are seen in their contradictory nature and are regarded both as forces progressing development and also as the starting point for pathological cementations.

   In contrast to family therapy, which sometimes tends to underestimate the importance of cemented mental and emotional structures, in psychoanalytic social work these and thus the *unconscious* needs of the client are given high priority. They are therefore registered not only in their positive valency as a resource for change but also in their problematic side, namely as a structural cementation.

2. This is accompanied by a stronger focus on the mental and emotional processes in the individual. For the purposes of illustration: many problematic psychosocial cases live in a social environment which seems to be keeping them where they are—in the case of an adolescent client this might be the parents. But let us imagine—as an experiment—blanking the parents out. If one did so, one has to admit that the problems would still be there, namely if one imagined the parents were suddenly killed in an accident, then, if not sooner, one would realise that the antisocial behaviour of the adolescent

would in fact continue to be as difficult as before even without the direct, further destructuring influence of the parents, which had been regarded—from the perspective of family therapy—as the crucial powerful negative influence.

This is an insight supported by experience and leads to a certain shifting of emphasis from working on the dynamics of the system to working on the mental and emotional structures, fears, emotions, wishes, and needs of the individual clients in order to change the relationship dynamics and so help the whole system to reach a state in which things function better.

## Milieu therapy and therapeutic communities

In its classic form milieu therapy, in the sense of a therapeutic community, puts its faith in the healing power of human community and as such has always formulated reservations about any form of therapeutic technique or exercising of social influence. In social pedagogy such approaches are widespread, beyond the relatively small sector of therapeutic communities, under the heading of *Lebensweltorientierung* or orientation to the client's world of everyday living. The healing power of the normality of everyday life is invoked, at times downright emphatically. In extreme cases a social worker with this approach may experience himself as the person who has to fight for and push through his client's participation in social life against an unjust distribution of social opportunities.

Here too, initially, there are important features we share: milieu therapy and therapeutic communities work to a great degree with the healing power of authentic relationships and these are also seen in psychoanalytic social work as being at the core of professional work. Frequently it is precisely the sense of reliability resulting from daily encounters and the growing understanding for the internal and external situation of the particular client that enable any kind of access to his world. Further, this kind of relationship in the everyday offers the client the chance to take on board something of what the social worker is offering and make it her own. Feeling understood and accepted, she can experience herself and her relationships afresh and this opens up new possibilities. Some severely impaired clients need such an anchoring of relationships in the everyday world in order to be able to let themselves enter into any relationship. We have described in another publication (du Bois & Gunter, 2000) the importance of infusing therapy intensively into day-to-day activities for inpatient treatment of adolescents with schizophrenic psychoses.

Ways in which psychoanalytic social work differs in its concepts from the therapeutic communities appear, above all, in the far greater awareness in psychoanalytic social work of the fundamental asymmetry of the relationships—here professional helper, there clearly impaired client. This finds expression also in the fact that the work of reflection on the emotional reactions of the social worker in supervision is given such importance. According to the understanding of the psychoanalytic social worker, scope for change opens up because the professional helper does not go along with the re-enactment of habitual, pathologically fixated relational dynamics but introduces variations, within the limits of what is possible and does not expect too much of the client (see Chapter Thirteen, Supervision).

The effect of this approach—in contrast to the views of the therapeutic communities—is an appreciation and the planned use of intervention and treatment techniques. These are not carried out in the spirit of some set intervention programme but are based on the social worker's constant reflection on his entanglements with the client.

## Socio-psychiatric interventions

It has long been known that psychiatric treatments of severe and longstanding mental and emotional disorders are hardly ever successful unless at least an accompanying social stabilisation is initiated and supported. Social psychiatry has developed on this basis and has produced a variety of forms. Today it is accepted as a matter of course that complementary educational psychiatric programmes are carried out for these patients.

Psychoanalytic social work, for its part, because of its therapeutic leanings, has always been actively concerned with mentally and emotionally severely ill and socially disintegrated people and has tried to develop specific forms of help for this group. So here, too, there are overlapping areas of concern and many forms of cooperation have been developed.

The differentiation is similar to that above for milieu therapy: in psychoanalytic social work interventions, measures, and programmes do not aim at seeing the clients settled in social institutions or integrated into social groups and structures. Rather, it seeks appropriate answers to the client's complex state of mental and emotional problems and the marked inability to cope with relationships that has often resulted from it. This often means that even those clients who do not fit into any of the standard care programmes can be helped with the aid of individually tailored measures to achieve social integration. Again and again it has been our experience that psychoanalytic social work with its individually attuned measures makes it possible in the end to integrate even particularly difficult adolescents and young adults with severe and chronic mental and emotional disorders in standard care social psychiatric or pedagogic institutions.

Psychoanalytic social work therefore works in a social area of complex structure between, on the one hand, therapy in its many forms—whether outpatient, semi-inpatient or fully inpatient care, psychiatric and/or psychotherapeutic—and, on the other, an equally varied field of social and educational forms of assistance.

Psychoanalytic social work is appropriate and likely to be helpful where mental and emotional conflicts and impairments play a role alongside social distress and cannot be successfully overcome by the corresponding psychiatric or psychotherapeutic methods of treatment.

A clear-cut demarcation, as is still sometimes common between social pedagogy and therapy and is not least encouraged by their completely different systems of financing, is in general inappropriate given the complexity of the problems and is particularly out of place for psychoanalytic social work, for this form of social work serves to fill a gap which, in view of increasingly shorter periods of treatment in the medical-psychiatric system and the structurally ever more complex problems in modern society, will continue to gain in importance.

## CHAPTER SIX

# Psychoanalytic social work and mediation

Mediation, which developed in the USA in the 1960s and '70s, is a form of settling disputes and conflicts in which an intermediary person, who is not dependent on either of the conflicting parties, works on a solution to the conflict that takes the interests of both into consideration.

Mediation is carried out in a regulated form; the preconditions are that the parties participate of their own free will, are capable of taking responsibility, and that they maintain confidentiality. The process does not aim at finding out supposed truths, determining a guilty party, or interpreting laws. Its aim is to set a process of problem solving in motion, maintaining self-determination in the solution of the conflict and bringing the process to a close with a consensual agreement (Besemer, 1993; Herzog, 2007).

As a rule the process of mediation is divided into five phases (Besemer, 1993, p. 15; Pühl, 2004, pp. 107 ff.):

1. Introduction—the parties make contact with the mediator
2. Working out the points of disagreement and views of the parties
3. Clarifying the interests and feelings of the parties and the background to the conflict

4. Working out ideas and options for solutions
5. Reaching an agreement.

This may be followed by a re-examination of the results of the agreement, possibly requiring a later correction.

Naturally, mediation as a way of solving conflicts through conciliation is not a new phenomenon in history. In a wide-ranging history of mediation, Duss-von Werdt (2005) assumes that conflicts are an anthropological given, that is, they are part of what it is to be human: they cannot be avoided but it is a question of "dealing with them in a civilized manner" (p. 20). His study is largely limited to Europe but he nevertheless points out in the introduction that conciliators are known to have been in existence in China for 6000 years. In Africa, too, forms of mediation are a part of tribal traditions and the "palaver" in its original sense is a "social institution of negotiation" (p. 20). Duss-von Werdt describes Solon as the first recorded mediator in European history. Solon was active as a mediator in the internal politics of Athens in the sixth century BC (pp. 24 ff.). A famous mediator whom he mentions at the beginning of the modern era was the Venetian Contarini with whose aid the Westphalian Peace was achieved (pp. 33 ff.). In one part of his book Duss-von Werdt goes beyond historical examples to collect and depict the range of the self-images of mediators—who saw themselves among other roles as philosophers, "trialogicians", partisans, fellow citizens, and democrats (pp. 145 ff.). This is a philosophical approach to the question of whether mediation is an integral part of everyday life in society or a professional activity. In the past a mediator carried out mediation as part of his wider areas of activity, Solon as statesman, Contarini as diplomat, simply because they were on the spot where a conflict had reached an impasse and had particular abilities in mediating. Today, by contrast, there is an observable trend towards the professionalisation of mediation.

Training to be a mediator is currently offered by many institutions. Some of them are privately funded but others are also under the aegis of associations and universities. In Germany the University of Hagen has correspondence courses in mediation in its programme and Oldenburg University offers contact courses for in-service training. Nevertheless the question remains as to whether mediation is "primarily a human attitude" (Geißler & Rückert, 2000, p. 41) exemplified in the "ability to tolerate conflicts" (ibid.) or whether it is a profession. The first view strongly advocates voluntary mediation (Metzger, 2000) while the second promotes a professional form of mediation.

There are many areas today in which mediation is applied. One that largely relies on volunteer involvement is community mediation, *Gemeinwesenmediation,* an area still in the process of being developed (Schulz, 2008). In very general terms the *Gemeinwesen,* in English more commonly referred to as community, refers to a form of organisation found in a group of people living in a certain locality but extending beyond the wider family. Today community tends to refer to a rather smaller local unit such as a parish or district in a town, but it can refer to the whole town.

Community mediation is concerned with conflicts between residents and administration, questions concerning the environment, intercultural conflicts, conflicts at work, use and design of public space, but also of conflicts between neighbours. Local residents function as mediators in this concept of community mediation: they are trained but work as volunteers. In doing so they may be working in the "stricter" or "wider" senses of mediation. Mediation in the stricter sense is concerned with concrete conflicts; in the wider sense it may be involvement in a larger structural issue concerning a whole district or over an institution such as a school, or it may be concerned with the longer-term participation of residents in the political life of the community.

In the final analysis, this concept of mediation touches on the growing disassociation of the administrative bodies from the people whose lives they administer. It aims at more participation and giving back responsibility to the residents themselves. One danger here is that mediation may be used as an adroit policy for smoothing over communal political-administrative conflicts: witness the fact that in some places there are plans to establish community mediation as a service in local government offices.

It is already a well-established practice in various legal processes, among others in divorce proceedings, in which a mediation leads to an agreement between the partners over financial questions and custody. A mediation is considerably more flexible than a court adjudication since the interests of both parties can be taken into far greater consideration without being subordinated to what are, as a rule, rigid legal prescriptions, and it is used today in many fields: in organisations it can be called upon in conflicts between the management and the works council, or over the merger of two companies, in team development within an organisation, or over dealing with bullying in the workplace (Pühl, 2003). For a description of mediation in a case of sexual harassment in the workplace see Haynes (2004).

In schools mediation is used to solve day-to-day conflicts and so increasingly pupils and teachers are being trained to act as mediators. The aim is not only to solve the specific conflict of the moment but to find a new culture of dealing with conflicts and disputes (Herzog, 2007).

## A theory of mediation?

Mediation is concerned with what action is to be taken. Accordingly, publications on mediation start straight in with a very detailed presentation of the principles of mediation, the mediator's interventions, areas of application, and examples from practice. Where there is any theoretical starting point, it is a theory of conflict. This is presented in relative detail in the literature on mediation by Besemer (1993, pp. 24 ff.; cf. also Kraus, 2005, pp. 35 ff.). In this description conflicts are ubiquitous and may be carried out destructively or constructively. In a destructive form the differing views of the problem are twisted into reproaches against the other person. The real problem is then no longer perceived, and instead the other person is seen as being the problem with the result that talking about the problem becomes more and more difficult, the parties reduce contact with one another, emotional entanglements increase, and so the ability to listen to one another or reach any agreement is lost.

If a conflict is played out constructively both parties look for a resolution without attacking each other. Instead of attacking, the parties take over joint responsibility for the problem and search for a solution. Thus they have a common focus outside their relationship to one another. Admittedly there may be many levels to a conflict, layer upon layer. Besemer speaks of four levels: those of the visible conflict, the conflict in the background, personality problems, and formative experiences from the past. If the last two are involved he sees a need for therapy rather than mediation. As examples of background conflicts in a conflict over an objective issue he lists the presence of different interests and needs, hurt feelings, disturbed relations with one another, different values, misunderstandings, and structural factors such as living too close together or too far apart, environmental factors, economic injustice, or political repression.

In mediation as described it is a question of finding new kinds of solutions for complex problems. The important new element here is the attitude of looking ahead to see what it may be possible to set up. In other familiar methods of resolving conflicts, such as arguing or negotiating, the parties are only looking at options for action that are already familiar and—as such—are not likely to lead to a solution of the conflict.

Besemer describes how in mediation the parties take over responsibility for the solution of the problems and conflicts. They learn with guidance from the mediator to refrain from using their competence, knowledge, and imagination to attack each other and instead share them to develop constructive solutions. Thinking in terms of victory and defeat is transformed into thinking harnessed to creating a shared solution to the problem.

For Götz and Schäfer (2008) the decisive instrument of mediation is language. They refer to modern theories of culture which regard the degree to which physical violence is replaced by language as a measure of civilisation. Referring back to Freud they emphasise that man can also vent his affect in words in the place of actions (p. 16). Mediation in this view is a process that makes people capable of using language.

## A psychoanalytic theory of mediation

Our reflections here sketch out a model for a psychoanalytic theory of mediation which for greater clarity is presented in the model of a conflict between two persons.

From the viewpoint of psychoanalysis human nature is constitutionally in conflict, the conflicts being rooted in the primarily instinctual and narcissistic constitution of human beings. The civilising of children's drive-driven needs and the surrender of their narcissistic orientation in order to turn instead to *objects* in their environment is forced on children in the course of their development in constant battles with the people in their childhood environment. Children learn self-control and renunciation in these battles and learn to be peaceable and caring. But the original renunciations and acts of altruism required of them only become part of themselves through internalising the experiences of relationships and so establishing mental-emotional structures. In this process the conflicts which originally took place in the external world are taken into a person's inner world. If this process runs without serious and lasting disturbances and impairments a person can achieve a balance between his or her own needs and the requirements of the external world. If, however, people have experienced serious disturbances in their development there is a danger that they will repeat the internalised painful experiences of their relationships later in their lives. This happens particularly when they have been affected in their narcissistic needs or when in the course of a regression their control of affects and needs is reduced, if, for example, *unconscious transference* elements of a failed early relationship creep into a current relationship.

Mediation is appropriate when the usual strategies for conflict resolution between two people have failed, leading to a long-term pattern of conflict. In the course of the conflict the other person has become a significant *object* with whom a dyadic, aggressively charged relationship has been established. Aggressive feelings are complemented by simultaneous, *unconscious* libidinous feelings in such a relationship and in order for a person to free himself from his own angry, destructive tendencies these are projected into the other person, possibly in the form of a *projective identification*. In the case of a projection, the other person is regarded as aggressive and angry and is treated accordingly; in the case of a *projective identification* the other person accepts the projective "offers", makes them his own, and behaves accordingly. In these mutual, malignant misapprehensions, and/or inductions of anger the libidinous hopes on both sides are constantly disappointed so that angry feelings multiply around the emerging fury over disappointment. And in the gyrating interplay of anger, hope, disappointment, and fresh anger both sides are focussed on each other and so incapable of standing back from the situation in order to reflect.

The mediator installs a triangular situation using the framework of the process and quite simply his or her own presence. In this triangle the predominant fears in the dyadic battle are spontaneously tempered: these are the fears of loss of self, of being overwhelmed or being destroyed by the other, and also therefore of the effect of a person's own anger. The tempering happens because the mediator is experienced as a protection against the destructiveness of the other person and also as a guard over the person's own anger. In a *splitting* of affects the mediator becomes the object of loving affects of both parties and this enhances his or her possibilities of influence. At the same time a mutual identification of the two antagonists with each other is established since they both love the same love object. The mutual identification makes empathic understanding of the other person easier. To receive recognition from the love-object (mediator) the opposing parties increasingly come to accept the steps he or she suggests. The opponent who is possibly the weaker one and more afraid feels protected against attacks from the stronger one and gradually dares to speak up for his or her own interests.

The beginning of a mediation process contains an unspoken, important message, namely.

"It is OK to have quarrels and quarrels can be resolved."

This *enactive/scenic* declaration, where the setup itself sends a message, triggers instant reactions and effects such as the release from *unconscious* feelings of guilt which are induced by the parties' own sense of "badness" over feeling anger and over quarrelling with each other. It is a dedemonising of their own anger which is no longer felt to be impossible to resist or world-annihilating but which now acquires a character of everydayness. And there is a lifting of the inhibition to speak up for their own separate interests since such representation of interests is legitimised.

The effect of all these processes, operating largely *unconsciously*, is that the parties can more easily recognise/accept and so control their own aggressive impulses. Through the tempering or ending of projective processes better reality testing can be achieved and with it solutions working towards an objective content become possible.

A case example is taken from the perpetrator-victim-conciliation service (Täter-Opfer-Ausgleich (TOA), Winter, 2004) which carries out mediation in cases of less serious offences. The mediation can replace court proceedings if both sides, perpetrator and victim, take part in the mediation and accept its results. TOA is a field in which it is helpful to work with staff who are sensitive and attentive to small signals which can often only be understood through observation of the staff member's or mediator's *countertransference*.

## A real-life example

The staff of TOA are given the task by the family proceedings court of mediating in a case of marital separation. The husband is alleged to have threatened the wife, to have intimidated her and their two school-age daughters and to have kicked down the door to the flat. All this is said to have happened after the wife had separated from him. He had moved into a one-room flat in the same building after the separation. After the incidents were reported he had received the injunction to move out of the building and not to approach his family for a certain period.

The husband was the first to be invited to talks with TOA and came across as a rather quiet, depressive, hurt, soft, professionally very successful academic, who had met his wife twelve years earlier. In his account she was quick to set about getting to know him and they had married after a few months. The wife had finished her studies but had not continued with her profession as the first child was born soon afterwards. A number of years after the birth of the second child she had taken training in a new field and finally, a year before the separation, had started to acquire a further qualification. In the course of this she had met another man and started a relationship with him. After a certain time she had told her husband about this and explained that she was separating from him. Since then she had shielded the daughters from contact with him on the grounds of his allegedly being a threat to them. The daughters had, however, he said, written to him to tell him that they missed him.

In the TOA interview the wife spoke of the threatening character, storminess, and violence of her husband after she had told him of her intention to separate. She talked of how she and the children were afraid of him. In the interview she showed herself to be a clever but cool and largely unapproachable woman. Of the daughters she said that they had no wish to see their father.

> In the psychoanalytic supervision the discrepancy was striking between the softness and understandable sadness of the husband and his alleged violence. Equally the impression made by the wife who came across as cool, somewhat manipulative, and well on top of the situation did not seem to fit with her alleged fear and helplessness.

Alerted by this discrepancy the view taken by the police and prosecution, namely "violent husband threatens wife and children", was challenged by the staff of TOA. In later interviews with both sides further indications emerged that the wife had clearly planned and coolly calculated her life, taking marriage and separation into her calculations. The violence of which the husband was accused was shown to be without real foundation. At this point suggestions were made for establishing in an appropriate manner what the children's interests were. The mediation process produced a restoration of the father's relationship with his daughters and an appropriate consideration of his interests in the regulation of the divorce, no longer influenced by the attribution of violence.

## CHAPTER SEVEN

# Psychoanalytic social work in day nurseries (day care centres), early education, and early intervention

Psychoanalytic social work for babies, toddlers, and preschool children supplements institutional early education and early intervention services as they have gradually been built up across the country or are in the process of being so. Above all, three areas are notable here in the psychosocial provision for families with very young children:

1. In Germany meanwhile there are some 1,250 early intervention centres across the country at present. Multidisciplinary teams provide in the main for babies, toddlers, and preschool children with disabilities or developmental disorders. These services are run by schools, socio-paediatric centres, institutions for the disabled, youth welfare services, and various charities. In the UK with Sure Start Children's Centres and early intervention centres it is similar.
2. Crèches and day nurseries for babies, toddlers, and preschool children. It is the avowed aim of the government to provide crèches throughout the country for very young children and this provision is gradually taking shape nationwide, though frequently with less than satisfactory conditions for the care of the children in terms of their psychological development.

3. In Germany the *Baby- und Schreiambulanzen* are outpatient centres for babies and toddlers offering counselling and treatment for infant sensory regulatory disorders, interaction disorders, and problems in psychological development in early childhood. Numbers of centres have risen markedly in the last few years, although one cannot speak of nationwide provision.

In the UK there is a cooperation between National Health Service and local authorities:

Local authorities run Sure Start Children's Centres with which NHS health visitors cooperate in accompanying families from antenatal care through to children at five years and can be among the first to pick up signs of disability, general problems of child rearing, and psychosocial problems—neglect or abuse. The NHS runs child health clinics and CAMHS, child and adolescent mental health services.

Alongside these, numerous counselling and assistance services exist for families with children, to which families with babies and very young children can also turn for help. In this heterogeneous institutional environment it has so far been hard for psychoanalytic social work to develop its own contribution or even a profile of its own. The areas of overlap are great and in this still young area of work for teaching and therapy a pragmatic attitude is prevalent according to which one copes with problems as they appear. This is also due to the lack of specialist services. Oddly, considering that psychoanalytic teaching has been intensively concerned with educational practice in crèches and nursery schools right from the start, psychoanalytic social work lacks an anchorage in these fields of work.

Psychoanalytic insights have been fruitful for educational work with children with both normal and disturbed development as well as those with other impairments. In the last few decades psychoanalytically orientated research on newborns and infants (cf. among others Dornes, 2000; Stern, 1992, 1998) has produced groundbreaking insights into mother-child interaction and the conditions that foster and encourage development or impede it in the care and upbringing of babies and toddlers.

Research on attachment, evidence on mentalisation, on self-reflective competence, and on control of affects (cf. Fonagy, 2001) has been widespread and its insights have been applied in counselling and educational work with parents of infants, toddlers, and small children, and also in educational therapy for this age group.

In most cases the early intervention centres see their central task as promoting the setting up of appropriate support for developmentally impaired and/or disabled children. Given this definition of their task they are frequently very much focussed on medical and functional aspects. Nevertheless, from the profile of these disorders it is clear that early intervention centres are confronted with not only the somatically founded developmental impairments but also with the wide variety of psychosocial problems and disorders in mental and emotional development which arise from them. As a result, in these areas of developmental problems they also offer counselling or arrange for it to be carried out by other agencies.

Children's centres also offer outpatient counselling and therapy services and may in particular cases offer inpatient mother and child therapies in cooperation with a clinic. They can be out of their depth, however, as soon as it is a question of complex psychosocial problem areas—which are often a central cause of the child's mental and emotional developmental disorders or of the interactional disorders between mother and child.

In all the overlapping areas described, in which the institutions named above are confronted with complex psychosocial problem areas, patterns emerge which require outpatient and follow-up social work to stabilise the family situation in order to create favourable conditions for very young children's development. This will, in particular, always be the case where parents are overwhelmed by the child's disorder and their own psychosocial problems and so cannot give appropriate care and attention to the child. What is needed in such cases is a form of social work which combines classic instrumental, social worker assistance with competence in developmental psychology and psychotherapy. The psychological burden on parents and the dynamics of the parent-child interaction can then be professionally supported. This represents a contribution from psychoanalytic social work that makes extremely good sense and has up to now hardly been used in early education and early intervention.

Although urgently needed, these fields of work have not yet been systematically developed. In such problem areas it is often a matter of chance whether and how the centres or clinics which are first approached arrange for outside professional help which can cover both the mental/emotional and social pedagogic requirements.

In cases in which cooperation has been set up, three forms of work have above all proved helpful:

### 1. Psychoanalytic social work with family and child in the home environment

Particularly when one or both parents succumb to mental illness, or there are ambivalently charged intra-family relationships, or the family is simply overwhelmed by the situation—then, besides counselling and support for the child's development the family usually requires the accompanying presence of a social worker. She can observe and address the disturbed interactions between parents and child and in the long run prevent an impairment of the child's development. Here, particularly, the parents will frequently be very ambivalent in their response, on the one hand asking for help, on the other experiencing any form of influence from outside as threatening.

The sensitive relationship between mother and child or between father and child is not sufficiently taken into consideration in support that takes the form of counselling, as in classic social work or in other forms such as may be offered in a children's centre with its early intervention concepts.

What is needed is an integrated concept such as is available in the framework offered by psychoanalytic social work. In the situations described above parents often already feel incompetent and devalued and offers of help seem to confirm this negative picture and further wound them. To ward off these feelings they declare the offers of help useless, a burden, unnecessary, or even persecutory.

It is often only after reflecting on these complicated dynamics in talking to the parents in an appropriate way that it becomes possible to set up a working bond and maintain it over a longer period as is needed for the stabilisation of the family. A service of this kind does not replace early intervention or counselling—it complements them.

### 2. Counselling for the institution over family dynamics, parent-child interaction, child's resulting difficult behaviour, and transferences to the institution

When charged interactional dynamics between parents over the child, or between mother and child, or father and child go off the rails, frequently these dynamics are rapidly transferred to the institution trying to help the family. One phenomenon is that families use the institutional services as a place in the "outside world of the institution" in which to stage conflicts they cannot deal with inwardly. This can happen in very different ways but it often leads to a situation in which the institution can no longer fulfil its real task but is completely taken up with securing the framework conditions and meeting an unending stream of demands, attacks, and problems in working with the family. At the same time, particularly in the case of children with developmental impairments, new symptoms are constantly presented requiring one treatment and intervention measure after another.

At this point the only thing that helps is understanding the underlying dynamics so that the institution can avoid beginning to act out, too, and can return to its real task instead. This necessary understanding of the dynamics can be achieved in different ways, for instance through a continuous counselling of the institution in the course of supervision or through case-by-case counselling. It would be beneficial for cases as difficult as these to set up either case conferences or a form of permanent counselling cooperation.

## 3. Psychoanalytic social work within the institutional setting

In specific cases with children who are hard to integrate it also makes sense, at least for a time, to have the child accompanied within the institutional structures with the aim of finally integrating the child in a special needs nursery school.

This form of psychoanalytic social work would see elements of direct work with the child combined with counselling for the institution and work with the parents. Because of the resources required it can only be considered an option for complicated cases with considerable impairments in social integration. It needs as a rule to be limited to a certain period, too, to be replaced gradually by one of the earlier-mentioned forms of psychoanalytic social work for families with very young children.

In view of the pre-eminent significance of the relationship dynamics between the main attachment figures and the child, for his healthy mental and emotional development, nothing is more important than detecting disturbances in the relationship early on. Disturbed relationships are mirrored in the interactions of the child with individual people and institutions. They easily produce an unreflected counter-acting-out on the part of the institution. This can threaten to undermine adherence to professional standards of treatment in the institution. Compared to almost any other approach, psychoanalytic social work is in a position to detect these processes in early education and early intervention for children and to develop methods of limiting the adverse effects of internalised relational patterns.

*CHAPTER EIGHT*

# Social work in real space and work on inner processes and structures

In psychoanalytic social work the tension between social reality, with which social work is concerned, and the inner world of thoughts and phantasies that psychoanalysis explores, is built into its very name. If we can keep the relation between internal and external reality well balanced and enjoy psychological health and flexibility then this opposition does not represent a serious problem. Quite the contrary it is, rather, a source of enjoyment when we consider what satisfaction and delight we can draw from the playful handling of phantasies when reading a book, for instance, or going to the cinema, watching television, attending a concert, or simply letting ourselves drift into private daydreaming.

This was what Freud meant when he wrote that a phantasy "is the fulfilment of a wish, a correction of unsatisfying reality" (1908e, p. 145). "Nevertheless," he wrote in another passage, "the mild narcosis induced in us by art can do no more than bring about a transient withdrawal from the pressure of vital needs, and it is not strong enough to make us forget real misery" (1930a, p. 80).

For many of our patients and clients, internal and external reality, far from being balanced are in conflict, often even creating a vicious circle with the reality of their lives a burden to them while their inner world is dominated by almost unbearable dynamics. They have been caught between a rock and a hard place and find it extremely difficult to find their way out.

Psychoanalytic social work is mainly concerned with patients whose inner state makes it hard for them to find their bearings in social reality. Their mental and emotional processes are no longer so flexible as to allow for a reasonably undisturbed adaption to the realities of life. These conflictual inner processes and the deficits in mental and emotional structures become so overwhelming that they cannot any longer be dealt with in the internal world alone. Instead they come out in pronounced *acting out*, plunging these people into one chaotic situation after another. In other cases the sometimes desolate social reality is experienced as so oppressive that it hardly leaves room for processes of inner development and working through.

A psychotherapy in the strict sense of the word, in which the conflictual inner problems could be guided towards a more beneficial solution, is unthinkable unless the external environment is stabilised and the problems with social reality are alleviated. Any form of therapy will have to involve these given external factors if it is not to miss the mark completely, ignoring the client's needs and possibilities and the way he experiences the world. In clients who need a setting of the kind offered by psychoanalytic social work one can observe various ways in which thoughts "spill over" into reality and reality into thoughts. Above all, two groups of clients can be distinguished here:

1. Psychotic and autistic children sometimes experience thoughts as if they were real objects in the room which then cannot be combined with one another. Thinking itself becomes reality to them; thinking of doing something is equated with carrying out the deed. Reality, for its part, is charged with symbolical meanings which can finally dominate thinking and acting. The real world, the world of objects is seen in symbolical equations (Segal, 1957) and becomes identical with what it means mentally and emotionally. Objects in this way gain a threatening life of their own and become as Bion describes it (1957, 1984) bizarre objects. These bizarre objects are combinations of an external *thing* and a part of the person's own psyche, and develop an uncontrollable existence of their own in his imagination. In the form of a delusion they can in this way become genuine persecutors. Thoughts and words turn into actual things in external reality and lose their function as symbols referring to *things*. 2. Clients with borderline personality disorders cannot

bear the simultaneous presence of opposite sensations and feelings. Others with whom they have a relationship have to be one-sidedly idealised. This idealisation collapses as soon as the shadow of a doubt is cast on it—for instance over a slight. The clients actively withdraw from trying to understand another person's behaviour by interpreting it, as would be natural, as an expression of the other's inner state and psychic processes. In this way their ability to recognise and understand in themselves the connection between *psychic* processes and actions is also endangered (cf. Bleiberg, 2001). Through pronounced *projective identification*, concern with the world of thoughts and feelings in the self and in other people is replaced by often destructive and autodestructive action in external reality, through violent interaction cycles in relationships with others.

Problems of this kind, in which mutual influence of internal and external reality results in a cementing of psychic and social problems, do not apply to individuals alone with their specific illnesses but frequently involve whole families, and here it is often hard to determine how exactly the external and internal problems impact upon each other and aggravate or further cement each other.

From its self-conception, psychoanalytic social work will always be concerned with the relation between outer realities of life and inner phantasies and so encourage a better connection between these two areas of reality through developing specific approaches for the clients and their problems. So, as social work, psychoanalytic social work makes a start with the client's real life world, well knowing that this is not failing due to the external conditions alone or because of the client's lack of strength and assertiveness, but also because here is a person who is forced to play out his inner conflicts in the social arena.

The psychoanalytic perspective enables an understanding of inner fractures not only in the *transference* relationship of the therapeutic one-to-one setting. It also enables an understanding of the complex *transference* and *countertransference* permutations that invade everyday relationships. These last affect and determine the interaction of the clients so much that purely educational approaches are often rapidly condemned to failure because they lack sufficient, appropriate, reflective, and thus distancing resources to counter an entanglement in malignant relationship dynamics.

It is only with the help of reflection on how psychic conflicts and incompatibilities in the inner life of the clients drive them to such actions that it is possible for the clients to return from a world of physical things, in which opposites often seem to exclude each other totally, to a world of thoughts in which different options can be allowed to remain alongside one another and in which therefore compromises become possible.

Admittedly, in contrast to patients who can benefit from a classic psychotherapy, for a long period and in many areas of their lives our clients need a psychoanalytic social worker to act with them in the reality of the everyday world to deal with the storylines they have developed. They need this person to react directly to their challenge and answer it in concrete terms in reality without losing sight of the story's importance in regulating the client's inner life.

A short vignette from the care and treatment of nineteen-year-old Andreas may serve as illustration. This is how it was reported to me in supervision:

> Andreas was preoccupied in his autistic phantasy worlds, among other things with monster-like, dangerous phantasy figures which had, on the one hand, very threatening qualities but which, on the other hand, protected him from the imponderables of life and the relationships associated with them.
>
> I learnt from his biography that he had been rejected himself, been seen as monstrous and dangerous, and had in his behaviour in adolescence actually corresponded to this image.
>
> Andreas had used practically all his savings to acquire a nearly seven foot tall plastic figure of a monster, in an auction. The monster was one of the figures from the fantasy stories which he used to people his inner world of phantasy.
>
> It was soon clear that what this young man was *bringing into his room* and thus displaying, was his self-image as a monster-like, dangerous ogre but also his desire for power and attractiveness. In German the expression *"in den Raum stellen"* is used to bring up or float an idea, that is, to make an idea visible, so Andreas was literally staging the German expression.
>
> The moment it arrived he took the figure up into his not so very large room and set it up there. It was important to him that all the carers should come and look at the figure and duly admire it. Though the immediate reaction of the colleagues was shock, this

was accompanied by a desire to acknowledge what he had managed to do and show appreciation of the importance of the figure.

While Andreas had long been able to talk about the figures of his inner world in therapy sessions he had up to then kept them hidden in his daily life in the group home and workshop. It was more than a year that he had been living there and with the carers he now had enough trust in the setting to dare to share something of himself and of how he experienced himself. He obviously hoped to find a place in the group home for this side of himself and, as I see it, unconsciously assumed that the staff, now being familiar with him, would understand something of the psychological relevance of this figure standing so dominatingly in his room.

Andreas had, moreover, weeks earlier told his parents that he had bought something really expensive. He made them curious but defended his territory by taking great care that they should not hear what this thing was.

The parents began badgering the staff of the group home, naturally wanting to know what it was, particularly since Andreas had told them that he had spent a considerable sum of money on it.

When the time came for the parents to visit him Andreas began to negotiate keenly with one of the staff on how to keep the figure out of his parents' sight. He was adamant that they should not see it. In order not to have to remove it from the room completely, just for the parents' visit, the staff member suggested heaving it up onto a kind of platform in the corner of the room which formed a sort of upper story where the roof sloped, and draping a piece of material over it.

In negotiating this in outward terms, using the concrete object he had bought and set up in his room, Andreas was also inwardly working on his desire for recognition of his inner world and his doubts that his parents would be able to recognise it appropriately—though that was what he longed for.

Finally the member of staff worked out a strategy with Andreas for exactly how to get this internal figure, which was filling most of the outer room, up into the higher part of the room, the *Oberstübchen*. In explicit terms it was about how to accommodate a large and awkward object that the parents were not to see. Implicitly and symbolically it was a dialogue about how an object in the real world, a great unwieldy thing, could be transformed into a thought. The German word *Oberstübchen* can also refer to a person's brain and mind.

This seems to me to be a characteristic example for psychoanalytic social work. Things have to be dealt with in concrete terms, they cannot simply stay in the symbolic space of language as would be possible in a psychotherapeutic setting. In therapy the focus would have been the story the patient told about such a purchase—not the purchase itself, and this story would have been related to the underlying dream thoughts and *transference* phantasies. Here, at the same time as he is negotiating over external concrete objects the psychoanalytic social worker is internally observing a theory of psychic development and relationship dynamics (Winnicott, 1971b, p. 7) that enables him to respond intuitively to the meaning at the *unconscious* level.

Thus, as Ernst Federn expressed it, it is not the task of psychoanalytic social work to turn social workers into "psychotherapists for the classes who can't pay so well" (1985, p. 25; quoted from Maas, 2004, p. 276). It is rather that in social work there are clients who cannot use their thinking processes in a way that might enable them to work in a classic psychotherapeutic setting and the task is to offer settings in which their inner situation is understood and so create spaces for thinking and relationship.

This means that in working with a client one is always working on the contradiction between the outer reality of life, for which there has to be room, and the inner life of phantasy which nevertheless creeps into social actions in daily life and embeds itself there. Psychoanalytic social work is therefore a kind of work on and in these intermediary spaces where thought-space and object-space overlap.

> Daniela had been sexually abused and prostituted by her father from nursery school age on. Beyond that she had for years lived more or less unsupervised on the streets but thanks to her intelligence was nevertheless able to manage at school. She was finally taken out of her family at the age of eleven and placed with a foster family.
>
> This family found itself in increasing difficulties because of her at times bizarre, at times unpredictable behaviour marked with outbursts of aggression. There was also the fact that she accused

foster father and foster brothers not only of sexual harassment but also the whole family of abusing and neglecting her.

At school—she attended a private girls' school which showed great educational understanding and engagement without which the task of accompanying Daniela through school could certainly not have been carried out—she became increasingly difficult and refused to occupy herself with anything but the things that interested her.

For example, for a while she was utterly fascinated by Thunderdome CDs, that were in fashion then, and dreamt up elaborate stories of how she was going to emigrate to Rotterdam and make a career for herself as a star dancer. Later these stories were replaced by a highly exaggerated identification with Africa, in particular with Mozambique, which dominated her entire thinking and experience to the extent that she not only dressed herself in clothes she sewed for herself in African style and collected Mozambique artefacts, but also sometimes indiscriminately approached people in town and talked to them about Mozambique only later to feel that she had been sexually pursued and attacked.

The extensive psychoanalytic social work with Daniela over many years had many facets. It began with her refusing any kind of therapy—"I am not ill"—and she was only willing to accept a sort of homework supervision to improve her school results. This took place several times a week.

In the course of this "homework supervision" the member of staff managed to make contact with Daniela—through negotiating the minimum needed to get through school as for any real work on the syllabus, there was no question of it. Africa played a central role over long periods.

She collected everything about Mozambique, drew maps, played strategy games with the member of staff in which she had to defend Mozambique, and was able in this way to stabilise herself fairly well and to function at school and in the foster family at least well enough not to be thrown out. Gradually over the years it was possible working with her to make a connection between the phantasy stories about Mozambique that dominated her thinking and her traumatic experience of helplessness, exposure, and impotent rage. She remained, however, dependent on a framework which could tolerate a good deal of her bizarre behaviour.

She had fixations which were sometimes aggressive, got out of hand, or crushed other people. Toleration for these was, among other things, achieved by carrying out continuous counselling on how to deal with them, not only for the school but also later for the trainers during her apprenticeship in an institution run on social pedagogic lines, and also for the foster family.

Daniela had previously acted out her threatening inner states to the point of making herself highly conspicuous and being perceived as almost intolerable, but over time she finally managed to give up this extreme behaviour. Meantime she is a young woman who may still wear dreadlocks, who makes her own African-looking clothes, at times with phenomenal skill, but who manages really quite well at her place of work and can maintain a number of stable social contacts.

The important thing in this casework was first of all to tackle the real conditions and accept that Daniela could only survive in a form of compulsively exaggerated staging of her extremely threatening and threatened inner state. Work with her had to start there and first of all stay in the external world and work on how to cope with that. Nevertheless the psychoanalytic social worker was always conscious of how much this *acting out* had to do with Daniela's inner world—and she experienced this in herself in absorbing almost unbearable emotional states when working with Daniela. Daniela was dependent on projecting everything into the external world that she could not work through inwardly, for instance in the "learning therapy session" this meant evoking these states of emotion in the psychoanalytic social worker in order, at least for a moment, to be free of them herself. It was only after a long period of work that this connection could be cautiously addressed. A client's *acting out* again and again proves to be an important form of *defence* which is to be regarded, alongside its pathological relevance, as a protective formation against unbearable inner states.

So, to a certain extent, *acting out* already represents a kind of attempt at healing and restitution which, however, leads to problems in reality. The necessity of *acting out* has to do with the fact that these clients often experience thinking and mental states as threatening, as something that leaves no room for other things. They cannot organise thinking processes as protective phantasies in the way we described these in the Introduction for the normal functioning of healthy people. They can only distance themselves from these inner states, which threaten to overwhelm them, by staging some element of them in reality (Gunter, 2000).

But this is precisely the great opportunity for psychoanalytic social work. Working with the client the psychoanalytic social worker can gently and tactfully try to translate back what was staged and accompany the client with understanding, helping him to develop other, less impairing forms of action.

## CHAPTER NINE

# Setting and adjustment of the framework to the needs of the client

I n psychotherapy and in particular in the classic, highly frequent psychoanalysis the setting, meaning the agreed framework conditions in which the therapy takes place, plays an important role. What is behind this emphasis on the setting is the fact that *unconscious transference* and *countertransference* processes can best be examined when sources of disturbance are kept to a minimum. As in a chemical experiment it is only in this way that reactions and counter-reactions can be reasonably reliably recognised and related to one another. A further reason is that the stability of the framework provides the patient with a certain basic sense of security needed for him to surrender himself more or less to free association. Whatever ideas and thoughts occur to him are to be censored as little as possible and not made to conform to socially accepted notions. For the analyst or therapist, for her part, the constancy of the external framework conditions makes it easier to maintain neutrality, empathy, and evenly suspended attention.

Psychoanalysis as a method of acquiring insight is essentially characterised by a form of reflection which enables access to the *unconscious*, but the great importance given to the external framework conditions for the proper and successful carrying out of a psychotherapy has led at times to psychoanalysis being commonly and in the popular view equated with certain settings and in particular with the high frequency of the standard treatment.

Freud had already pointed out in his volume, "Lines of advance in psycho-analytic therapy" (1919a) "that the various forms of disease treated by us cannot all be dealt with by the same technique" (p. 164).

He was convinced that psychoanalysis contrasted with other methods of therapy not so much on the basis of its specific therapeutic technique and the framework conditions associated with it as above all by its method of acquiring insight.

Psychoanalytic social work treats questions of setting and framework conditions in a completely different way from that just described for psychoanalytically orientated psychotherapeutic work. In contrast to the psychoanalytic procedures, which prescribe a clear setting for treatment, in psychoanalytic social work, after careful reflection, the framework conditions are systematically adapted to the *unconscious* conflict patterns of the client. The decision for flexible adaption is based on the observation that it is precisely those in need of the kind of therapy that psychoanalytic social work offers who cannot or cannot sufficiently fit into predefined frameworks. They first of all have to establish relationships in real space and experience relationship structures that differ from those with people (*objects*) they have so far known and internalised (cf. Chapter Eight). To enable them to do this the framework conditions have to be adapted in such a way that they do not ask too much of the patient as regards intellectual capacity and ability to deal with affects.

This means that the setting is not, as is usual in psychotherapy, a prescribed, only slightly alterable element. Psychotherapy and psychoanalysis offer with their defined setting a space for the development of psychic inner life; psychoanalytic social work, by contrast, aims first of all to create conditions of any kind that will make an external space possible and with it a psychic space for thinking (cf. Bruns, 1999).

This means that the question is always: what does this or that form of care, this or that combination of forms of help, this or that frequency of contact mean to the specific client consciously and unconsciously? What conflicts will possibly be triggered by an appointment? What conflicts are excluded by a choice of setting?

In this way it may be necessary, in one case, to contact a client daily and visit him several times a week, irrespective of whether he is actually there at the agreed time or prefers to be somewhere else. It may be extremely important to him—irrespective of his general state at the time or of his attacks on the relationship and his verbal outbursts—that someone should show reliability in a way he has perhaps never experienced in his life up to this point.

Another client might experience precisely this setting as encroaching on her space or persecutory, since she feels herself constantly under surveillance and regimented by an inner *object*. A client such as this would presumably benefit more from being able to ring up the outpatient clinic or the home group whenever she felt it was necessary and ask for advice just about everyday questions. Whether she would make use of the advice would be left to her.

Such flexibility in handling setting and framework conditions means not only that individual setting constructions have to be invented for different clients but also that the setting has to be adapted in the course of care to the current state of the client's inner dynamics.

This means not only applying the stages, quite usual in social work, from full inpatient treatment to assisted living and from there to occasional socio-pedagogic help when it is needed. What is meant here is a far more systematic adaption of care to the *unconscious* dynamics of the client (Kraft & Perner, 1997), right down to tiny details of the framework. There are innumerable examples of adapting very individually to particular clients of which a few may suffice here:

It may make sense at first to visit a family one is starting to work with twice a week to convey to them that they are respected and that one is interested in the circumstances of their life. The feeling of shame and devaluation and the resulting aversion to any educational measure were so great in one particular family, because it was connected by the parents to traumatic experiences of devaluation in their families of origin. There came a time, however, when one of the children was asked to come to the outpatients department for some of the sessions by bus. This was to support a development towards greater independence which was desired but also feared because it departed from habitual structures of conflict.

The child's efforts at a transition to independence were torpedoed by the mother because of her own denied desires for detachment, so that as things went on it became necessary to offer *her* sessions in which she was able to talk about her lost childhood and being worn out with caring for her parents.

A young man of seventeen was admitted to one of our home groups after he had "failed" in several institutions. At first he could only accept the idea of being admitted to a home with "these disabled guys" when offered intensive training for a prospect of work. This training also offered him the chance to escape a desolate family situation, but although he was capable of fair intellectual perform- ance his cooperation was unconsciously subverted by provocative behaviour. He was caught in a conflict between his bond with his mother, an emotionally unstable alcohol dependent who exploited him mercilessly, and his desire to detach himself from her. He trans- ferred this conflict onto the group, putting the fear of God into them and trying to undermine the authority of the carers. His pathologi- cal identification with the mother drove him unconsciously to get further and further into debt by taking out contracts for one mobile phone after another, but on actually getting the phones he handed most of them over to his mother and other close relatives.

Having his own flat—although intensive support of him continued—defused the situation. At first, visits by staff from the home group were daily with the goal above all of keeping up mini- mal standards of order and cleanliness in the flat.

A central theme was for a while the question of whether really all the available electrical equipment, from TV to stereo set to electric fire and computer, had to be kept on at the same time. Gradually he was able to talk to staff about the psychological meaning of this waste of electricity and permanent bombardment with sound.

Parallel to these conflictual themes he was advised by another member of staff in weekly sessions about dealing with his debts. She was not otherwise involved in this case but alongside her work as psychoanalytic social worker she was in charge of running the institution as a whole.

The debts were listed systematically and paid back according to a readily comprehensible plan. This specific relationship was something to hold onto and had a structuring function that went far beyond the outward question of regulating debt. It addressed the central questions so important to him of the reliability of *objects*, their kindly attention and availability, though also their *triangulating* setting of boundaries. Thus a third principle came into play, so to speak the position of the father, limiting his pathological attachment to the mother and establishing reality in its rightful position.

Finally the setting changed again. He concentrated his contacts on fewer people and was able to say far more clearly how important staying in the institution was for him. In one-to-one therapy he began to have thoughts, although sometimes in a rather bizarre manner, about the relationships that were important to him in his life and about their meaning. He was not well able to bear being visited in his own flat at this stage but regularly kept in contact with the home group, coming over often for visits and was very pleased if after staying away for two days he received calls asking how he was. Right down to small details, such questions of the setting can become significant for the course of the work with the client.

Nine-year-old Manuel had, for certain periods, been taken out of his family on the grounds of neglect and placed with a foster family. His mother informed us that she had hated him from the start but she nevertheless wanted to have him at home at all costs. Manuel was allowed to go back on condition that the family members declared themselves willing to cooperate in sessions with a psychoanalytic social worker. The agreement was that Manuel should also be examined at the child and adolescent psychiatry clinic to assess whether they could answer for letting him stay at home in the given circumstances.

At first the fundamental distrust the family showed was in the foreground. Intensive talks with the parents gradually enabled this to be reduced. The examination at the clinic led as agreed to the writing of a letter of recommendation to be submitted to the local authority children's and young people's services. Now the mother's distrust was directed against the recommendation—which had in fact been discussed with her—that not only was there to be counselling for the parents but a separate therapy for her. The mother complained to the psychoanalytic social workers who were carrying out the sessions with both parents and she demanded this should be changed.

The child psychiatrist who had examined Manuel in the clinic insisted on having a further meeting to discuss this, which involved a certain delay. In the end mother and father both came to this meeting and here the mother was able to make her point the subject of discussion: she wanted recognition that the father, too, had an important function in the family.

The presentation of the boy—as requested—at the child and adolescent psychiatric clinic helped to "disperse" a little the paranoid basic attitude of the family and so to stabilise the cooperation in the framework of psychoanalytic social work. Through changing the setting to give it a more imposing character it was possible to make the seriousness of the situation clear to all, at the same time, however, as limiting the scope of the mother's manipulative tendencies and thus temper the repetition of paranoid ways of experiencing linked to them.

So with these clients alterations to the setting are frequently as effectual as interpretations in classic verbal psychotherapy. These changes in the setting take up aspects of the *unconscious* structure of the client and, if the *unconscious* dynamics have been well reflected on and are appropriately introduced, they can act on the client as an impulse to reflection and change.

Verbal interventions do not generally have sufficient effect on this clientele (see Chapter Five) and are often and for long periods rejected as "just talk". In their orientation to the symbolism of actions and language verbal interventions do not appear to have enough weight for these clients. They seem intangible and indeed incomprehensible to them in comparison with interventions on the level of actions and settings. One could call the latter "interpreting via deeds".

Flexible handling of the setting with its adaption to the *unconscious* dynamics of the clients also often means that complex setting constructions are required. The various forms of intervention have already been briefly outlined in Chapter Four. It is often remarkable how the various functional relationships of the different members of staff (e.g., support in communication with the authorities, help with integration in the workplace, work with the parents, etc.) can give rise to very different *transference* dynamics so that there is a chance for the clients to get to know the various facets of their own personality.

When one is aware of this range of *transference* options provided by offering different relationships in the setting, and understands this as part of the therapeutic educational possibilities of psychoanalytic social work, it becomes clear that the clients not only present themselves but also become aware of themselves in the various areas as in varying degrees competent or impaired.

Flexibility in handling the setting should not, however, be confused with arbitrariness, or an attitude of "anything goes". It has to be accompanied by constant reflection on what one does and be based on abstention, empathy, and neutrality. Abstention here does not mean leaning back and thinking things over, for in any individual case the situation will call on one to act. Reflection will follow. To ensure abstention it is important not to confuse one's own interests with the task one has taken on: namely to help the client to achieve the greatest possible development and capacity to live and maintain relationships while allowing oneself to be guided by the client's ideas.

## CHAPTER TEN

# Transference—countertransference— "scene"—the enactive domain

In psychoanalytic treatment the *transference* of the analysand and the *countertransference* of the analyst are the most important paths of access to the *unconscious* of both participants. Both are important in psychoanalytic social work, too, but here a further path to the *unconscious* is added which has already considerably enriched the classic concept of *transference* and *countertransference* for psychoanalytic treatment. In psychoanalytic social work this path acquires even greater weight on account of the enactive dialogue between carer and client: it is scenic understanding.

## Transference and countertransference

Freud introduced the concept of *transference* as an element of psychoanalytic treatment in the depiction of the case of Dora (1905e, p. 115).

> It may be safely said that during psycho-analytic treatment the formation of new symptoms is invariably stopped. But the productive powers of the neurosis are by no means extinguished; they are

occupied in the creation of a special class of mental structures, for the most part unconscious, to which the name of "transferences" may be given.

What are transferences? They are new editions or facsimiles of the impulses and phantasies which are aroused and made conscious during the progress of the analysis; but they have this peculiarity, which is characteristic for their species, that they replace some earlier person by the person of the physician. To put it another way: a whole series of psychological experiences are revived, not as belonging to the past, but as applying to the person of the physician at the present moment.

While it is true that Freud had already used the term *transference* in "The Interpretation of Dreams" (1900a, p. 561) he had, however, used it there to refer to a process of displacement in which an *unconscious* thought merges with a harmless, conscious idea, perhaps some memory of the day, and can so make its way into consciousness. But with the publication of the Dora case, *transference* appears as a regular element of psychoanalytic treatment. Freud goes on to say (1905e, p. 116) that the psychoanalytic treatment does not in itself create the *transference* but merely uncovers it. A few years later he differentiated between positive and negative *transference*, or the *transference* of tender and of hostile feelings (1909d). During treatment, he wrote, various, at first diffuse, feelings towards the analyst might develop and apply to the whole analytic situation, an effect Freud referred to as the *transference* neurosis (1914 g, p. 153), in which all the patient's symptoms would have taken on a new significance in the framework of the *transference*. In this way they had become accessible to therapeutic work and thus curable. At the same time the *transference* can become a *transference resistance* as in the form of *transference* love (1915a). Nevertheless a mild positive *transference*, an "unobjectionable" *transference* seemed to him to be a helpful, motivational force for treatment (1912b, p. 104).

Perceptions of *transference* underwent considerable development after Freud (see Herold & Weiß, 2008). The two essential elements which mark post-Freudian understanding are the consideration of the analyst/analysand relationship and the experience in the here and now which depart from Freud's paradigm of the nature of *transference* as intrapsychic and as being exclusively a repetition. These aspects were already discussed by Ferenczi and Rank (1924).

With the concept of *projective identification* (Klein, 1946) and its further development in the *container-contained* model by Bion (1962a), *transference* becomes part of an essentially *unconscious* exchange relationship between analyst and analysand to which both are indispensable contributors. Winnicott, as the representative of British *object relations* psychology, links the contribution of the analyst to the development of an atmosphere conducive to treatment and therefore to the patient's *transference* in the concept of the *holding environment*, analogous to the *holding environment* for a child's development (1965, 1971a). In self-psychology, too, as developed by Kohut (1971) in the treatment of narcissistic disorders, the necessity for the analyst to have an attitude of empathy towards the patient is emphasised. It allows the development of twin and mirror *transferences* which show the patient's use of the analyst as a *self object*—according to Kohut this is an essential stage in such treatments. *Transference* becomes even more radical in the social-constructivist view as something negotiated between analyst and analysand to which the analysand initially provides a contribution in the form of his neurotic *compulsion to repeat* (Gill, 1984; Hoffman, 1991).

After the use of psychoanalytic treatment was extended to include psychotic patients, psychoanalysts discovered the *transference* psychosis in analogy to the *transference* neurosis (Mack-Brunswick, 1928; Searles, 1963). In the *transference* psychosis the analyst is built into the patient's psychosis: the patient loses therapeutic ego *splitting* and with the loss of reality testing he can no longer distinguish between *transference* phantasies about the analyst and the analyst's real behaviour. He is convinced that this is what the analyst is like and that he is behaving in the way that is attributed to him. The *transference* psychosis can become an insurmountable *resistance* in treatment.

After the discovery of *transference*, phenomena of *transference* began to be noticed outside the therapeutic situation. In present-day perception, *transferences* take place in all human relations in which a particular significance is attributed to the other. In its most general form *transference* simply means that particularly in difficult and frightening situations people habitually turn back in their feeling and thinking to the relational models that they know—and these are the early *object relations*. Doing so offers them the advantage of a certain security and orientation but can also have the serious disadvantage that they cannot judge the current situation realistically. They experience this, rather, as a familiar earlier situation, analogous for instance to situations in childhood relationships. It is always elements of internalised *object relations* that are transferred to the *transference* object. Preferred, common objects of *transference* are persons such as teachers, clergymen, doctors, police-men, partners, own children, and colleagues. It can also be people beyond the closer circle of acquaintance such as politicians, film stars, or sportsmen who become the object usually of an idealising or devalu-ing *transference*. And not only individuals but also organisations can be chosen as *transference* objects: from football clubs, social services, and local authorities to charities and even states.

Freud mentions *countertransference* for the first time in 1910, saying it was evoked in the physician "as a result of the patient's influence on his unconscious feelings" (1910d, p. 143).

The physician should recognise this *transference* in himself and mas-ter it. A psychoanalyst, Freud wrote, could only do as much as his own complexes and inner *resistance* would allow. He must begin his profes-sional work with a self analysis. With reference to *transference* love he spoke of the necessity for the physician to contain or "hold down" his *countertransference* (1915a, p. 163).

Although he had initially felt it to be a disturbance, Freud grew to use *transference* more and more for psychoanalytic treatment and later saw it as a powerful aid in the treatment. *Countertransference*, however, remained in his view a disturbing element to be kept down and moni-tored in order to maintain the attitude of impartiality, free of personal interest deemed desirable (ibid.) in treatment.

This view of Freud's has undergone the most far-reaching expan-sion and alteration of all Freudian concepts. Laplanche and Pontalis (1973, p. 164) point out that through the application of psychoanaly-sis to new areas such as analysis of children and psychotics, in which more demands are made on the *unconscious* reactions of the analyst, and through a changed perception of psychoanalytic treatment, which has increasingly become understood as a relationship, the concept of *trans-ference* has changed. They present two opposing views: one regards anything of the analyst's which may intervene in the treatment as *coun-tertransference* while another regards the analyst's *countertransference* as his response to the *transferences* of the analysand.

In the first, wider interpretation, there should, strictly speaking, be a distinction drawn between an analyst's *transference* to the patient and his *countertransference* response to the patient's *transference*. Möller

(1977) specifies afresh the classic view that *countertransference* is the non-neurotic reaction of the analyst to the patient's *transference*.

An important step for the further development of the concept of *countertransference* came from Helene Deutsch (1926) who distinguished between two attitudes the analyst had to the patient's *transference*, a complementary attitude and one that identified with the ego of the analysand. Racker (1959) combined this distinction with Kleinian theory and reached a distinction between a concordant identification of the analyst with the ego and id of the analysand—for example with his sexual wishes or aggressive reactions—and a complementary identification of the analyst with the inner objects of the patient (p. 73). The analyst must learn to perceive these intersubjective and inner processes by *splitting* his ego into one that experiences and one that observes, corresponding to the therapeutic ego *splitting* required of the patient (Sterba, 1934).

Racker's reflections build here on Melanie Klein's ideas concerning the way unbearable psychic states are constantly conveyed to a significant other, particularly from child to mother with the help of *projective identification* (see Chapter Thirteen). Similar ideas on *countertransference* were developed by Paula Heimann (1950) in her assumption that in *countertransference* the analyst's *unconscious* understands the *unconscious* of the patient. She states that the *countertransference* is created by the most pressing elements in the *unconscious* of the patient—and can therefore be regarded as a mirror of these elements.

Finally, Bion (1962a) extended this concept with his *container-contained* model in which the infant conveys to the mother, as described in *projective identification*, the unbearable and uncomprehended elements of its inner life—the as it were undigested feelings and perceptions which he referred to as beta elements. The mother, for her part, undertakes the digestion of these beta elements by modulating them into alpha elements which are bearable and comprehensible for the infant. She then gives them back to the infant in this form. Alpha elements in Bion's terminology are the psychic contents which, in contrast to raw sensory perceptions, can be digested with thinking and feeling and so be turned into narrative. With this work a decisive process of exchange for the infant's psychic development is described. The description can now also be taken as a model for the perception of the processes between analyst and analysand.

The further developments of the concept of *transference* and *countertransference* have given formulation to the current perception that psychic life is determined by intersubjective processes. *Transference* and *countertransference* cannot be separated from one another; the one emanates from the other.

Intersubjective processes can remain completely on the psychic level but can also merge into interaction. Sandler (1976) postulates that, at least in certain circumstances, an element of interaction can be interposed between the patient's *transference* and the *countertransference* reaction of the analyst. This expresses an "intra-psychic role relationship" (p. 300) not as yet verbalised in which the patient casts himself in one role and assigns the corresponding complementary role to the analyst. This *role relationship* can express itself in action or enaction and will in some cases only be understood after the event. The concept of *interpretive action* created by Ogden (1994) is based on a similar idea. Here it is the analyst who acts and in doing so gives the patient an interpretation—though he himself at that moment may well be *unconscious* of its meaning: he acts on the basis of a *countertransference* reaction which is not as yet conscious or understood. Exchange processes of this kind also take place in the relationship between social worker and client.

## "Scenic" or enactive understanding

In 1970 two Frankfurt psychoanalysts, Alfred Lorenzer (1970) and Hermann Argelander (1970) published articles on scenic understanding (*szenisches Verstehen*). By the word *Szene* they mean the way an analysand shapes the psychoanalytic situation. Earlier experiences of relations and psychic relationship representations enter into this "shaping". This means that in the treatment situation patterns of internalised *transference* and interaction are *unconsciously* played out in an enactment.

The first psychoanalytic interview already offers the patient considerable space in which his *unconscious* psychic constellations may be expressed. But it is particularly in longer-term psychoanalytic relationships that *unconscious* relationship representations make their appearance. Here consciously intended efforts to shape interpersonal dealings retreat and through the patient's mild regression, induced by the familiarity with the relationship, already existing *unconscious* patterns of relationship come more to the fore.

In any relationship one can observe that the behaviour of the participants is consciously controllable so long as they are still relative strangers to one another. The closer and more familiar they become, the more the plannable surface of behaviour melts away and the more the core of a relational behaviour, which cannot be consciously controlled, makes its appearance. This core is built on *unconscious* relationship patterns internalised at an early stage. This is what happens in psychoanalytic treatment and, as we see, in social work.

Argelander (1970) assumes that the ego with its "scenic" function enacts *unconscious* infantile configurations in a manner adapted to the situation. Perceiving this allows the analyst to grasp an *unconscious* conflict beyond what can be understood via words. In Argelander's view the part of the narcissistic libido which is not permanently bound by sublimation or the building of character formations is available for the enactive representation of an *unconscious* conflict.

Lorenzer (1983) substitutes the concept interaction for the reifying term thing-presentation. To memory traces he gives the name *situation representatives*. He is referring here to Freud's differentiation between word-presentation and thing-presentation. Word-presentations are closely connected to language and therefore to the conscious; thing-presentations gradually come into being earlier, before the child has developed a command of words/language but experiences the relation with the mother as an interactive relation. In modern neurobiological terms this is the differentiation between the implicit (*unconscious* preverbal interactive) memory and the explicit (more conscious, narrative) memory. In this way a non-verbal layer of symbols is seen to exist beneath language symbolism. The psychoanalytic process revolves around the axis of *transference* and *countertransference*, that is to say the psychoanalytic relationship. Thus with this *scene* or enactive representation an interactional experience achieves expression which, because it had formed before the development of word-presentations, could at first only be communicated in a scene or an enactment. Interactional enactment is seen as one stage. A further stage is understanding the images as in dream and, finally, naming what the enactment is about completes enactive or "scenic" understanding.

Klüwer (1983) took these ideas further by combining them with Sandler's (1976) concept of the *unconscious* role relationship. Subject and object play roles with one another in therapy, too (cf. Winnicott, 1971a). The enactments of the patient are seen as "invitations to the therapist to take over the unassigned role in the cast" (p. 833). In this way an enactive dialogue develops and in his view it is a present-time actualisation of the *transference* and *countertransference* in the form of the patient's acting and the analyst's acting-with-him. As a result the so-far-*unconscious* interrelating roles can enter consciousness.

### *Transference, countertransference, and Szene—enactive representation—in psychoanalytic social work*

The concepts of *transference, countertransference,* and "scenic" under-standing were developed in psychoanalytic treatments with their defined setting and their deliberate distance from the everyday. The psychoanalytic situation is characterised by its framework (Bleger, 1966) and by a method of self-reflection, that is, by the free associations of the patient. For the analyst an essential element in the method is his oscillation between identifying and distancing, between experiencing and interpreting. Framework and method create a third presence in the situation to which both participants refer. In this way a triangle is pro-duced which enables reflection on the situation, that is, the third angle enables the participants to observe the treatment and the processes in it from an excentric position outside what is happening and from there to reflect on meanings.

The social worker is face to face with his client in an everyday set-ting. He or she has no situational structure aiding reflective distance to the client and the situation—as the analyst has to his patient—but on the contrary is involved in it to a great degree in action and reac-tion. The client is encountered in direct interaction frequently marked by heavy "transference pressure". This transference pressure grows out of the disorders or illnesses of the client of psychosocial work. In the main these are the so-called early disorders which are linked with early *defence* mechanisms such as *splitting* and preverbal forms of communi-cation. In the intersubjective field, processes of *projective identification* predominate. In these, near intolerable affects and phantasies are ousted to be located in other persons. Inner conflicts are often not played out and solved on an inner stage but are acted out in actions in the exter-nal world. Therefore it is enormously helpful if staff take note of these enactments and realise that they contain a communicative significance even if this is not immediately comprehensible.

Since the external interactions and the psychic exchange processes take place directly and very rapidly, psychoanalytic social workers have to be able to a high degree to tolerate tensions, intense affects, and projective ascriptions of affects to them. It is all the more important that social workers should have the opportunity to talk over these interactions outside the field of work in a protected space, and so be able to speak about their experiences, fears, and the overwhelming nature of demands made on them. This is their "triangular" structure allowing reflection on the situation and their relationship to the client. A space of this kind is to be found in regular and timely supervision. Supervision produces a protection against situations in which entanglements get out of control and conflicts escalate (see Chapter Thirteen).

## Example case 1

A young patient was born into a situation where she was unwelcome to both her parents. The mother was still young and was living on her own, while the father was married to another woman. When he left his wife two years later he moved in with the patient's mother but the couple separated again very soon. For a second time the patient experienced living alone with her mother. During these years the mother often left the flat at night after the patient had gone to sleep. So, waking and finding herself alone, she would run over to the neighbour's and wait there in tears for her mother to return. When she was five her parents reunited and lived together again for two years. After the next separation her mother took her to see her father at set times, dropping her off at the door and driving straight off. The father was often not at home and she would have to wait hours for his return.

This patient developed a psychosis at the age of seventeen. Three years later, after repeated spells in hospital, she began a psychoanalytic treatment. She cannot stand being alone. Sometimes she wakes up at night and feels panicky fear when she realises she is alone. She usually sleeps at a boyfriend's. She is filled with the fear of being unwelcome and cannot bear it if her mother doesn't agree to a visit. When they do meet she can't leave and makes her mother almost desperate. She also can't let go of the analyst after sessions. At first she just remains sitting in the consulting room. On being spoken to repeatedly she makes her way out into the corridor and stays there for a while, sitting on the floor.

In the *transference* the analyst has become the mother who left her alone at night and dropped her in front of her father's door. To avoid the unbearable feeling of being abandoned she refuses to leave the analyst after sessions, virtually clinging to him. In the *countertransference* this triggers in him a feeling of being pestered and constricted. He also has the impulse to get rid of her which is similar to the young single mother's urge to shake off her overly clinging daughter. In the treatment, however, the patient finds a different solution by working through the fears of separation and abandonment.

## Example case 2

Nineteen-year-old Albert, living in a group home, is presented in supervision (Gunter, 2006a). The carers depict with considerable affect the way he besmears and messes everything up. They have been getting terribly angry with him. If one asked him to take green waste to the compost he would come back a minute later having obviously thrown it into the general waste. He claimed however that this *was* a bin for green waste which made them so angry they felt they had to go to the bin with him and put the green waste onto the compost with him—thereby virtually encouraging his muddle-headed behaviour. They would really like to tell him to do this on his own but he wouldn't be able to do it.

Similar scenes were played out over clearing up after eating together. When this was his job everything was left in chaos and was mucky. He had knocked over the Christmas tree a number of times. He had completely messed up the kitchen, throwing everything including plastic, meat, and other food into the organic waste bin so that maggots collected there. At times they felt he was doing it to provoke, at other times they knew he didn't know how to behave in any other way. And he was eating them out of house and home, tucking into five portions of everything. Then again he had to be specially called to the evening meal. Recently he had practically run into one of the staff and nearly knocked her over: he said afterwards he had urgently needed to go to the kitchen to fetch himself a spoon for the spaghetti. In the incident he had jumped up and run straight "through her". He had simply stormed out regardless of who was in his way. He had also virtually wrecked his room. Initially he had set up his room very tidily, meticulously and installed his furniture, put down a carpet, and arranged everything nicely. But recently they had found what was probably urine in his apple juice.

What is known from his previous history is that his mother had from the very first found him repulsive. The father was mostly absent, but would turn up from time to time, unannounced; he would hit the children, give them orders to behave themselves, and then disappear. He is said to have had relationships with other women. The mother too was chaotic and was herself without any supportive relationship. Up to the moment of this report she was still in this state. If he was at home at the weekend she would ring up and complain that he was terrible and that she couldn't bear him any more. If she was offered a structuring or reduction of his visits to her she was against that too.

From these scenes with Albert—which not coincidentally centred around food—it is possible to infer an inner *object* and relational world dominated by chaotic, contradictory, and unpredictable *objects* destroying all order. In his everyday relations, affects—which he cannot deal with in thought and thus integrate with the help of an alpha function—are *enacted*: a scene is created. Chaos serves the function of a *defence* against these affects, the mechanism being to scatter things. If his inner world had any order these affects would come up against *objects* (i.e., internalised people), but this would be frightening. So the member of staff, a woman, is not attacked directly as the object of his anger and hatred but his attack has the appearance of a chance happening, the side effect of a sudden hunger driving him to the fridge and he simply mows down everything in his way. The affects are not thought over, integrated and controlled but first of all discharged in actions in his surroundings.

It is only with an understanding of this situation on the part of the carers that affects and happenings are given a meaning which would not be gained by "training" or "teaching" him. He showed similar behaviour, an acting-out that created chaos, in the accompanying one-to-one therapy.

## CHAPTER ELEVEN

# Cooperation relations in psychoanalytic social work (interagency working)

Psychotherapy, and most particularly psychoanalytically orientated psychotherapy, takes place in the relationship between therapist and patient. Influences from outside are seen as disturbance rather than as part of the therapeutic process. Strict confidentiality is maintained except for a very few exceptions even as regards family. The work of therapist and patient centres on the inner processes of the patient. Anything emanating from outside enters only through the subjective view of the patient to figure in the therapeutic exchange. This attitude has only changed with the increasing numbers of the treatments of patients with severe disorders who are also in a tangle of problems of social integration and are dependent on social support in a variety of forms. Professionals began to acknowledge that influences on therapy from outside and interventions of the therapist in the social world of the patient's life could be an important element in the therapeutic process.

By contrast social work has always been grounded on a self-conception that sees work in the social field as its main task and as a result regards relations of cooperation with other institutions, providers of aid, authorities, and the social environment as a crucial part of their task.

This was further accentuated by the focus in the modern practice of social work on orientation to the client's living environment and social field. There is, however, a danger here that dedicated action in the social field becomes equated with improving the outward situation and the social competence of the client and that current practice may advocate the limiting of interventions to what is material and instrumental. This can mean that psychosocial problems are not seen in their true complexity.

There is no doubt that most of the families, children, adolescents, and young adults who require social pedagogic care depend on a functioning connection and cooperation with other systems of support. It often falls to the lot of social workers and pedagogues involved to set up access to other services for their clients or to mediate in the frequently erupting conflict situations between institutions and clients or institutions with each other. And so social work needs to have a concept of cooperation with other and often differently structured help programmes. In reality such reflections have hardly been developed: for example, there may be the requirement for someone to be on hand in the long term to help adolescents and young adults with addictive disorders and to coordinate the help programmes whose implementation is long overdue. Even such quite generally formulated requirements regularly fail for lack of professional structures and financial resources. Furthermore, the central importance of properly functioning cooperation lies in its being able to create access to places to live and supportive relationships for more severely impaired clients. The areas such as support for living accommodation, for work, and therapeutic one-to-one care are so separated off from one another that they are used and experienced very differently by the client, but in fact they need to be connected to create an overarching concept that fosters development. Interestingly, it has been observed that in these different life contexts clients can sometimes develop very different levels of functioning in their inner, psychological organisation and in their social functioning (Gunter, 1994 ). The deliberate breaking up of institutional structures with the transitional spaces that emerge for clients at the same time requires work on a stable basis for cooperation.

Psychoanalytic social work can contribute to establishing a theoretical foundation and to the practical implementation of such cooperation structures. This is because in psychoanalytic social work people with their conflicts and the kind of needs they have move into the main focus of attention where they are seen not only for their conscious but also in their *unconscious* problems. The activities of institutions and help agencies, and the measures taken, for their part, are always reflected on in terms of what conscious and *unconscious* needs they address and satisfy in the client and what conflicts they activate or diffuse. This means there tends to be a shift from regarding measures solely in terms of their outward and objective function of support to ensuring that the subjective aspect is always included. Namely, this subjective aspect has the power to cause the failure of technically well-designed measures. Psychoanalytic social work with the accompanying reflection on the often complex and variously fragmented *transference* relationships consistently tries to examine and understand help systems from the viewpoint of the client and the expectations he unconsciously harbours.

This has a number of consequences:

1. It can be assumed that many of the clients being cared for perceive the institutions concerned with them both realistically and at the same time distortedly through the lens of their emotional expectation. In this way the local authority and the children's and young people's services may be seen realistically as a caring institution but at the same time can be perceived as controlling.

   On the other hand, however, this authority may be met with childlike needs for nurture and care which, part consciously, part *unconsciously*, determine the client's relationship to the female member of staff concerned.

   If claims are rejected, this desire for nurture and care may suddenly switch to anger which is projectively warded off through paranoid fears of being persecuted by the youth care services. If one recognises and understands these connections one can take an empathic stance towards the family concerned and understand their needs and neediness. This can help one not to side too completely with the family against the authority concerned. One also possibly avoids the opposite reaction of seeing the family as uncooperative, exploitative, and deceitful even if they show a few tendencies in this direction.

2. Many clients have marked idealisation and devaluation tendencies which are often transferred to the various institutions and persons working in the help system in the form of *splitting* processes. In a case where the local authorities have assigned two people to help a

family, it can happen that the family idealise the "help" who drives the client to go shopping—using her own car to do so—while the case manager is regarded as having something against the family and as persecuting them. And he may, for example, be accused of just looking for reasons to take the children out of the family into care. The psychoanalytic social worker who is a newcomer to the case is forced from the start into seeing things in black and white: either he allies himself with the family as a friend or he appears as their opponent on the side of the authority which is experienced as threatening.

The recognition of such *splitting* processes and an understanding of the inner conflicts from which they result can be a first starting point for finding a mediatory position which takes the fears and neediness of the family seriously while naming the worry felt over the unsatisfactory provision for the children.

3. Importantly, what is gained by applying such a reflective attitude is being able to see the *splitting* processes as inner psychical reality that needs to be taken seriously and as attempts to cope which command respect. This approach can prevent things coming to an unreflected polarisation of positions between care agencies. For example, in the shared care of *splitting* clients or patients a social worker and a psychiatrist may come to clash: the psychiatrist, who has been asked to examine a worked-up, paranoid, and aggressive patient, sees, on examining the patient, no such signs and cannot understand the social worker's assessment: the patient, she says, is perfectly reasonable in the way he talks to her and she does not need to be told how to do her work, above all not by social workers who understand nothing of the matter. The social worker, who has sent in the patient for examination, is insulted and angry over the psychiatrist's lack of understanding, her lack of appreciation of the dangerousness of the situation, and her argument, limited to medication, that the patient is receiving enough neuroleptics.

Such clashes show how the patient keeps the different aspects of himself meticulously apart, indeed must keep them apart, in this way carrying the *splitting* of his inner world into external reality since an integration would be too dangerous to his inner mental and emotional balance. To do so he uses the boundaries between institutional structures. This form of *transference* can take on the dimensions of a *projective identification* in which those involved as objects of the *transference* become so infected with the corresponding projections of the patient that they can no longer distance themselves or free themselves from the *unconscious* attributions.

If such processes are known and recognised there can be ways out of dead end situations of this kind in which otherwise the patient and the institution concerned become helplessly and usually destructively entangled.

4. The psychoanalytic reflection described leads to a new situation in which the different measures and help programmes, the different institutions concerned, and the locations at which the patient is supported are connected. In this situation they are not simply added together without any inner consistency but all interventions are reflected on continuously, keeping the total effect of the interventions and their meaning for the client in view.

To use an image, one could say that a symphony requires the concerted effort of the whole orchestra; it is not the effect of a single instrument that is the focus, as can be the case in a modular approach.

Many factors have to be considered and balanced. How much can the client *integrate* and what will cause *splitting*? How to balance recognition of his neediness with perception of his own resources and needs for autonomy? How much to support him and how much to demand from him? These questions all need to be incorporated in the practical execution of an overall support measure if a situation is to emerge which is reasonably bearable for the client and in which he can cooperate.

It is essential to prevent single measures or the type of relationship from reactivating conflicts and fears that are unbearable for the client. Such reactivation would, possibly, drive him into aggressive, oppositional *acting out* which would cause the failure of the measures intended to help him.

5. This leads us to a further significant fundamental of psychoanalytic social work.

If one takes seriously the fact that the way relationships are set up in the socio-pedagogic field is of great relevance for the activation or diffusion of inner conflicts, then the logical consequence is that measures should not only be planned and put into practice with outward goals in view but must equally be set up with the development of psychic structures and stabilisation of unstable conflictual patterns in mind. Thus institutions are required to show considerable flexibility and willingness to adapt to the psychological structure of the client. If an intervention does not function in the way it was planned the first question should be to what extent it was perhaps incompatible with the *unconscious defence* structures of the client and whether it might have triggered fears which the client could only keep at bay through *resistance*.

6. Also from the point of view of the planner this means that any later changes such as adapting the intensity of a measure, the target agreement, the structuring, or the framework conditions must always be reflected on in terms of their meaning for the client.

> In the case of an adolescent girl in supported housing, for instance, an increase in the frequency of visits, designed to prevent her sliding into self-neglect and to step in before the flat becomes completely run-down, is experienced by her as unbearably controlling. *Unconsciously* she may be connecting to a mother who, on the one hand, never really looked after the child and, on the other, paid meticulous attention to keeping everything spotless, tidy, and presentable. Increasing the number of visits would possibly exacerbate the conflict and lead to marked counter-reactions. It might even speed the downward development into neglect and endanger the apprenticeship she is up to now regularly pursuing.
>
> An alternative in a case of this kind is to invite her to join in cooking a shared lunch with others of her age and a carer in the outpatient day care centre.
>
> Beyond that one could reach an agreement with her to have a weekly visit from a member of staff to her flat where they would share the cleaning up and have tea together. If the assessment of her inner dynamics was right she would not have to develop so much *resistance* as in the first variant.

Looking ahead, Chapter Twelve is dedicated to the most extensive cooperation and intensive coordination with children's and young people's services and/or other funding bodies, and here brief notes are given on the other partners with whom cooperation over support is most frequent.

## Integration in school and workplace

Often one of the underlying causes of the need for extra help is that the school can no longer cope with certain children or adolescents. Not only does this mean that their development is considerably impaired

but also that they are threatened with losing important social relationships and contacts. So it is a part of the social worker's task to keep
in touch with the school and offer counselling. In particular cases the
school needs direct support so that the child or adolescent can continue
at school and not have to be excluded. Some children and adolescents
need special schooling which is tailored to those suffering from mental
health problems.

In our clinic, for example, we have set up a one-year course pre-
paring for work that offers five places for adolescents suffering from
mental health problems and an annex of the clinic school for children
and young people with autistic psychotic disorders. Frequently such
pupils cannot find appropriate schooling in schools specially designed
for children with behavioural difficulties or in schools for children with
mental retardation.

The cooperation with the school has to be so set up as to make a clear
divide between the area of schooling geared to external reality and the
educational therapeutic area which brings in the pupils' inner reality.
This is, as a rule, possible even with severely impaired children and
adolescents and sometimes leads to surprising stabilisation in one area.
However, such developments cannot readily be transferred to the other
areas.

Adolescents and young people with mental disorders often have the
greatest difficulty fitting into work structures. Even in social enterprises
or similar programmes for the disabled they are often initially in need
of extra help as their problems are of a particular nature. To have a psychoanalytic social worker to mediate in this process has proved very
useful: accompanying the client to the workplace for certain periods
and complementing sessions with the client by talking to the responsible teaching staff in the institution.

In this way it is often possible to avoid over-challenging or under-
challenging the client. In working with adolescents it is important in
a particular case to make clear what is typical adolescent behaviour,
which can be difficult for an institution for adults to cope with, and
what can be traced to mental and emotional problems. This differentiation allows for more appropriate responses. Sheltered work institutions
(social enterprises) for difficult adolescents are often over-challenged
when expected to assess such disorders correctly. They do not have
experience in using appropriate ways of dealing with them as they
more often work with youngsters showing externalising behavioural
disorders.

## Specialists in psychiatry

Setting up good cooperative relations to consultant child and adolescent psychiatrists and consultant adult psychiatrists and also to the locally responsible hospital is very much to be recommended. Often it is crucial in a crisis situation to be able to fall back on such relations and also to have clinically competent partners at hand. It is to the advantage of a psychoanalytic social worker team to know and accept pharmacological methods of treatment.

In working with hospitals whose staff are not very familiar with psychodynamic thinking a lot of tact and skill is required to ensure that psychoanalytic understanding of a case is taken into consideration in setting up the plan of treatment. One should not launch into long-winded explanations of the client's psychodynamics. Rather, what is helpful is pointing to the acute psycho-pathological symptoms such as states of excitation or paranoid ideas. Often the patients need the hospital to find a few days of rest and detachment. The patients and the doctors treating them in the psychiatric unit need the opportunity to talk to each other. Nevertheless it can be very useful if a key carer also speaks to the doctor, best of all in the presence of the patient. Such a person can describe the problems and conflicts from the viewpoint of the group home.

## Other agencies involved

Cooperation with other agencies of social work for children and young people demands particular tact in certain cases. When psychoanalytic social work is set up in addition to the previously installed measures of support these social workers can often feel slighted. Conflicts are often sparked over the question of how far any change and improvement can be achieved if measures are limited to instrumental help—which is perhaps seen as "blind actionism" from the point of view of psychoanalytic social work. From the other point of view, the social worker working already with the family may see the analysis of the relationship dynamics between herself and the family carried out by the newly-arrived psychoanalytic social worker as condescending and know-it-all. The danger here can be that *splitting* processes emanating from the family will be taken up and exacerbated by this situation of competition and rivalry.

In such cases the following is recommended: on the one hand to reach agreement with the local authority on clearly delineated remits but on the other hand also to try to set up a common supervision. A successful solution in many cases has been to regard the existing measures set up by the local authority as part of the external reality of the family or client, as the case may be, and for the psychoanalytic social worker to deal with the institution in a friendly, neutral manner. Sometimes, however, handling double sets of care measures can be so complicated that the only thing that helps is to decide for one measure or the other.

## Justice system

As with psychiatry the relationship of social work to the justice system is not without tensions and problems. But if one works with adolescents and young adults who have come into conflict with the law one should not underestimate the boundary-setting and thus stabilising function of judicial procedures and sanctions. There are adolescents with whom one can only build up a relationship if this is an order made in their probation sentence by the court. In this case the duty to report on their development is to be regarded as part of reality with the help of which a certain framework is created.

It has often proved disastrous to diverge from such framework conditions for what one regards as good educational reasons and to set up one's own private laws. Looking the other way out of friendliness in the hope that the situation will be diffused or that things will calm down not infrequently produces the opposite of what one desired and carries the danger of positively triggering an escalation.

So, in working with young people of this kind, one will always have to deal with their search for a boundary-setting object (person or institution), which according to Winnicott plays a role in every case of antisocial tendency. The tussle with this boundary-setting object is to be seen as a sign of wishing for a relationship and therefore as a sign of hope (Winnicott, 1984).

## CHAPTER TWELVE

# Cooperation relations with the institutions carrying the costs of social work

Measures involving psychoanalytic social work are as a rule funded by local authorities, specifically children and young people's services or social services. In the course of formal procedures—such as setting up a care plan—the making of necessary arrangements and other forms of cooperation may sometimes appear time-consuming and irritating and can lead to many differences of opinion between public and private support agencies, which can sometimes make appropriate and client-orientated decision making harder. Nevertheless one should not underestimate the opportunity this formalised procedure offers for psychoanalytic social workers to explain the dynamics and problems in the case to the local authority social workers in particular, in a way they can understand.

There is here a difference, extremely hard to bridge, between a perspective which is primarily concerned with outward, tangible, and, in extreme cases, actionable need for support and a way of viewing the case which makes the inner dynamics and relationship dynamics of a family the yardstick for the planning of interventions. This difference poses considerable problems in reaching understanding.

To avoid the misuse of this genuine structural difference to create incessant arguments, what is first of all needed is for each side to acknowledge the form and content of the other's. It is the right and the duty of the local authority services to examine and check the necessity for a measure and to reach a professional, well-founded decision. For this the psychoanalytic social worker, for her part, needs to present and give reasons on the basis of her specialist knowledge for her assessment of the need for help, and to explain alternatives and risks. Experience shows that her views with their supporting arguments are often taken up as supportive by the locally responsible social worker and taken into consideration in the decision.

Cooperation can fail if there is fundamental rejection of psychoanalytically orientated work or if, from the start, commitments have been made to other approaches to understanding cases and taking action in this field. Questionable, insufficiently objectively founded rejections of aid measures are above all to be found at the next level at which decisions on cost absorption take place. Here professional arguments are at times subordinated to economic constraints.

At the outset and in the course of every assignment it is established practice to provide the public agency funding the measure with the necessary professional explanations so that they can reach their decisions on costs. Usually the responsible local authority social workers are glad to receive competent, understandable reasons for a measure to support their evaluations. Beyond this there is a legal requirement to write reports in cases of risk to the well-being of the child.

The situation makes heavy demands on psychoanalytic social workers. Alongside showing professionalism in their work they have to be able to describe complex relationship dynamics, a *transference/countertransference* pattern, and inner conflicts and, moreover, do so in terms that non-specialists can understand. These intra- and interpersonal processes can often only be indirectly deduced. To make them understandable and transparent for a colleague who is not familiar with psychoanalytic thinking is not always easy.

One has to bear in mind that psychoanalysis often meets with a mixture of idealisation and devaluation. On the one hand it is invested with the aura of an occult science capable of penetrating into matters deeply hidden and ready with explanations and solutions for the most difficult situations. On the other hand it is declared to be out of date and out of touch with reality and little or no notice is taken of the major developments in psychoanalysis that have taken place in the last decades in theory, technique, and the practical aspects of treatment.

This ambivalence towards psychoanalysis makes it particularly important in reports and exchanges with colleagues not to strike attitudes of superior knowledge but rather to translate one's insights into the "everyday" language of social work in a pragmatic, case-based, understandable, and approachable manner. A report is only helpful if the person receiving it really has a chance to visualise and understand the results of the work process so far and be able to examine it critically. If there are uncertainties in an assessment these should definitely be pointed out and not covered up with the use of psychoanalytic jargon. There is an opportunity here, for instance, to make it comprehensible why a family or client cannot accept the well-meaning offers of help which are actually perfectly in accord with professional standards. Working with examples can illustrate what inner problems prevent the family from accepting help. This makes their refusal understandable. There might be, for instance, a conflict with authority which is instantly activated when a social worker approaches the client though she does so with the best of possible intentions. Or again it could be the client's *unconscious* deeply-rooted feelings of absolute worthlessness which make him experience an offer of help of any kind as a slight and a humiliation no matter how much this offer seems to make sense and be perfectly tailored to his needs. In view of the uncertainties in social work mentioned in part above it is often hard to produce a positive, forward-looking description of what needs to be done and what has been achieved while remaining aware of the limits of what one's professional actions *can* achieve.

Sometimes the problems of a family and their background are hard to assess. In such cases a probationary phase of care has proved helpful. In this phase better insight can be gained and measures can be developed that are more appropriate in form and length. Frequently the local authorities will request this measure with corresponding expectations. What is important in this context is that the time limit of the probationary phase is clearly and openly named and explained to all concerned, including the family, and that this phase is designed first of all solely to evaluate the situation. It serves to sound out the concrete shape of help needed and to develop ideas on how to set up the measure. There must be clear agreements about the extent and timeframe of this phase and these must be communicated to the family, too. During the probationary phase the children involved may, however, develop intensive relationships which—if the phase were to go on longer—could not be interrupted without affecting them seriously. In order to avoid fresh, painful experiences of relationships for them such phases should be kept as short as possible, especially when it becomes clear they will be discontinued. In the course of psychoanalytic social work meetings take place with the parents in which they talk about their own biography and general mental and emotional state. In these, as also in the thera- peutically orientated one-to-one sessions with the children, the clients can talk very openly about their own problems, often a matter of shame, and about their psychic conflicts. These conversations touching on very personal areas are often comparable to the discussion of personal prob- lems in psychotherapies. Such openness is only possible if clients know that what they have told the psychoanalytic social worker and their internal relationship to him or her will be reliably protected.

On the other hand it is the duty of such a social worker to report on the progress of the measure to the authority funding it. He or she is also expected to inform them of new problem manifestations only now emerging in these sessions. Dealing with this situation, in which necessary confidentiality conflicts with the duty to report, requires sen- sitivity and tact. In a specific case, one has to weigh which elements are essential out of the information confidentially conveyed and consider what is important for the process, and which details are possibly deci- sive for the dynamics but dispensable for the report to the public fund- ing authority.

If there is trust and reliability in the cooperation with the public funders it may make sense to discuss details of the client's problems in a framework that includes all involved.

We ourselves have occasionally found it helpful to invite members of the local authority children's and young people's services or social services to our supervision sessions. On the other hand the distrust of public institutions felt by the families involved and their fear of inter- ventions must be acknowledged. There may sometimes be violent disa- greements with them over this, but informing the clients about the duty to report to the local authority services is nevertheless an important clarification. Then one can discuss with them what is to be included in the report.

The same applies to the reports themselves. They should be written so that nothing is whitewashed but that they can still be read by the clients. This demands a great deal of sensitivity, clarity in stating one's own view, and the courage to state it. It is a question of addressing problems in a manner respectful to the client but nevertheless stating the case clearly. Possible effects of the report need to be considered beforehand. If objections are raised later by clients it is then necessary to take them seriously in the light of their *unconscious* dynamics and incorporate this in the further process. Sometimes such objections, absurd though they may seem, provide pointers to inner conflict dynamics one had up to then overlooked or they offer the chance to talk to clients about so far excluded fields of problems and conflicts.

In work orientated to therapy the care plan itself can also produce considerable problems. One thing is the danger that the client feels he is alone, confronted with a majority of professionals he perceives as hostile, and experiences this as a betrayal of the emotional relationship established with the social worker.

Another is the frequent experience that in such discussion of the care plan for them clients follow their need to appear as normal as possible. They minimise their problems and neediness, which can endanger the extension of the measure. Such situations may place the psychoanalytic social worker in a very difficult position because pleading for an extension of help measures also means making the client's deficits clear, which he may experience as a slight and as devaluing him. Uncritical confirmation of his abilities would, however, be to his disadvantage. It might give him the satisfaction of a short-lived narcissistic confirmation but it would bring about the ending or reduction of the aid measure. This too should be discussed with the client beforehand. It needs to be clarified in these sessions with the client where he himself sees the need for help and how he would like to argue for it. Further, the client has to be told the view the social worker is going to present on the case. It should also be pointed out that one not infrequently experiences the opposite situation, in which having the client take part in the planning process makes it extremely obvious to the responsible social worker at the local authority how necessary the measure continues to be.

In presenting what has been achieved so far it is important to make sure that there is a clear and understandable connection between outward and visible changes in behaviour—social or work integration, improvement in parenting competence, social stabilisation, starting into work—and processes of inner change and development. This connection has to be clear in order to demonstrate what specific approaches in psychoanalytic social work have been followed with a successful result. Only in this way will the authorities be able to understand that there may be a need to support a further stabilisation, even though goals in the external world, for instance integration into work, have been achieved. Conversely if *not* much has changed in the outward social situation of the family by making the correlation between inner and outer situation clear, inner developments can be highlighted. As has been described in the previous chapters those involved with clients are often entangled in complex *transference* and *countertransference* processes. In the course of this, negative affects are often projected onto social workers working for the local authority. They come across as persecutory, malevolent, intrusive, unfeeling, and cold, which is not only a source of great strain but can lead to understandable but unhelpful counter-reactions.

As a psychoanalytic social worker one should be very careful in the emerging *splitting* processes in such situations not to take too "literally" the idealisation of the one side and the devaluation of the other. This does not mean one should not be aware of their seriousness and of the powerful effect they have on the perception and behaviour of the client. One should, however, learn to understand such distortions as a *transference* manifestation of the client's problems with an inner conflict.

It is often helpful in the communication between the various different institutions, particularly between local authority services and non-government agencies, to reflect on such *transference* expressions and examine them for the consequences they produce for care planning. Colleagues in local authorities are grateful when reflection of this kind makes them realise that they have become the objects of *transference* phantasies attributing malignant and persecutory intentions to them. But it can also happen that the psychoanalytic social worker finds himself in the position of the persecutory object; this, too, should be disclosed.

In a different therapeutic context I myself (M.G.) have frequently experienced how severely ill children suffering from life-threatening diseases in the oncological ward of the children's hospital have projected everything negative and malignant onto me when I was called in as psychiatric-psychotherapeutic consultant. They could not show all their hatred and their despair to the paediatricians and nurses looking after them or to their parents. But the children dared to show these feelings to me and it was at least a relief for a while in their existentially threatening situation. My difficulty was how to get it across to the colleagues on the children's ward that this negative *transference* was important for the children's mental and emotional balance. I had to put a brake on the tendency for the colleagues there to attribute every burdensome and negative development in the children to me as if I were really a threatening monster upsetting their children.

Psychoanalytic social workers also sometimes find themselves in a similar situation when for a time a negative, paranoid *transference* cannot be resolved but is decisive for the progress of the work and for the development of the client. It is helpful then to inform others involved in the case and explain to them the dynamic function of such a complex *transference*. In particular with *projective identifications* such a *transference* can lead to local authority support workers and the family becoming hopelessly entangled and even to the support workers losing their professional distance. Tact is demanded here in order to convey the possibilities of reflection and understanding to be drawn from psychoanalytic social work in such a way that this is perceived as support for the colleagues and not as instruction, or a patronising know-it-all attitude or arrogance.

Given the complicated relationships in social care, truly anybody can be caught up in the whirlpool of *transference* and *countertransference* dynamics that initially resist reflection. This is no reason for casting doubt on the competence of a colleague. On the contrary it is a good opportunity to rethink the problems of the client, taking the *transference* as a starting point, and to work for a deeper understanding. Where there is *resistance* to self-reflection, however, this is unlikely to be achieved.

*CHAPTER THIRTEEN*

# Supervision

S upervision is indicated and in many cases indispensable everywhere that people work with people and where relationships between people are an essential part of the work. This includes the entire psychosocial area, education from child care to schools, and the whole area of care of the sick. Beyond these it is applied in hierarchical fields of superiors and subordinates and in teams of colleagues on an equal footing.

The need for supervision stems from the fact that we all have a tendency to allow our own very particular mental-emotional disposition—made up of our fears, expectations, and current state—to influence our professional relations with other people, in this way following our *transferences*. This can lead to serious misapprehensions, false interpretations of situations, or entangled interactions. Situations of this kind may considerably impair a person's ability to work. Supervision can help to understand such situations and find solutions for them.

The Swiss professional association for supervision, organisational consultancy, and coaching (BSO) gives the following general definition of supervision: "Supervision is intended for individuals and groups or teams of staff. It concerns itself with concrete questions arising from the everyday professional world of the participants and also with questions

133

of cooperation between people in various roles and functions, areas of work and levels of hierarchy. It is the aim of supervision to improve the working situation, working atmosphere, work organisation and competence related to specific tasks. It is designed to foster practice-centred learning and the quality of cooperation" (quoted from Belardi, 1998, p. 44).

Supervision has two historical sources. One, rather older, is social work in the United States of America. Originally volunteer staff working in social service were guided and counselled by full-time professional staff. From this setting there emerged a kind of guidance and help that was linked to specific cases. The guidance was at the same time combined with a controlling-supervising function (Möller, 2001, pp. 17 f.). The other source was the supervised analysis in the framework of training for psychoanalysis candidates set up in 1920 at the Berlin Institute of Psychoanalysis (ibid., p. 18; see also Roudinesco & Plon, 1997, pp. 565 f.). The carrying out of "control analyses" has since become a regular part of the training for the profession of psychoanalyst worldwide.

## Foundations of supervision

Whereas the aspects of guidance and control were in the foreground with both the supervision of social workers and of analysts in training, since then, with the wider applications of supervision, further aims have developed. Supervision is not only used in psychoanalytic and psychotherapeutic training or in the psychosocial field but also in administration and in profit-making organisations with their emphasis on yield. Supervision is expected to give counselling on complex tasks in human resources, institutional infrastructure, and communication in organisations. Alongside increasing work efficiency it is expected to help prevent burnout in staff and carry out crisis intervention and innovation consultancy (Möller, 2001, p. 13). With these new tasks, supervision has itself undergone further development from being a supervision of training to supervising the everyday work of individuals, teams, groups, and institutions.

In the early days of supervision psychoanalytic concepts formed a foundation of understanding (Steinhardt, 2005, p. 22), not only in supervisory analysis but also in casework supervision in the USA. They have remained a decisive element of practically all approaches to supervision, as a glance at overviews of the literature shows (Möller, 2001;

Pühl, 1999, 2000). However, other theoretical elements have been added corresponding to the extended area in which supervision is applied. The most important are group dynamics and the sociology of organisations. For individual areas, such as the psychosocial, teaching, and the profit-making, particular approaches have been developed which, alongside the knowledge of process dynamics drawn from psychoanalysis, group dynamics, and the sociology of organisations, include knowledge of subject matter in the corresponding field.

Federn, one of the pioneers of psychoanalytic social work, describes two forms of supervision, one in which "the supervisor only has to understand how to carry out supervision" (1994, p. 15), and the other, as in American social work, where the supervisor is teacher and superior, that is, knowing more about the field of work than his tutee. He regards a combination of the two forms as the best solution: the supervisor "should have great experience in the field of work being supervised and also be expert in the process of supervision" (p. 16).

## Psychoanalytic supervision

Supervision can be carried out in the form of individual supervision or group supervision. In group supervision it may be a group which has only met for supervision or a group that works together permanently, often a team (team supervision). In individual supervision, as a rule, the aim is a better understanding of the case and therefore the attention and focus of interpretation lies in the case being presented. In team supervision it can be more a question of the team dynamics, as for instance when the team's ability to work well is being considerably impaired by unresolved conflicts.

From the supervision of psychoanalytic treatments Engelbrecht (1990), for instance, describes "how the psychoanalytic situation is enacted in the supervision", how the analytic situation being presented is relived in the supervision session. Scenic understanding enables a broadened understanding of the psychoanalytic process. This understanding should, however, only be used to understand the patient and not for an analysis of the conflicts of the colleague concerned (p. 679). Bauriedl (2001) describes "scenic processes of change in supervision" with individuals and groups.

As in all relations between people, *transference* and *countertransference* stemming from the "here and now" of the supervisory situation will also emerge between supervisor and supervisee. This plane is enriched, however, by the fact that mirroring phenomena manifest in the supervision: the relations between a physician and his patient or between a psychoanalytic social worker and his client will be mirrored in the supervision, with the supervisee taking over the position of his patient or client and the supervisor that of the supervisee in the treatment or care situation. The "then and there" in this way becomes the "here and now" (Kutter, 2000).

One model of the *transference/countertransference* relationship in supervision is Bion's model of *"container-contained"* in which the supervisor, as the container, transforms the uncomprehended beta elements of the treatment into alpha elements for the analysand (Lazar, 2002: see also Chapter Ten in this book and *container/contained* and *projective identification* in Glossary). The pattern for this model is drawn from the relationship between mother and baby in which the mother carries out this process of transformation and conveys the content back to the baby in more digestible form.

In psychoanalytic group supervision it is mainly three psychoanalytic group models that come into play:

- The Balint group, which was first developed by Balint in work with general practitioners. In this model the group serves to mirror enactively or scenically the *unconscious* conflicts of a presented patient or of the doctor-patient relationship and/or makes these easier to grasp through the stimulus of the *unconscious* of members of the group manifesting in the verbalisation of ideas which occur to them (Loch, 1995).
- The Bion group model which starts from the oscillation between two states in the group, that of the working group and that of the regressive basic-assumptions group. In the basic-assumptions group characteristic, fundamental conflict patterns appear: dependency, fight/ flight, and pairing. In the supervision group the regression of the group to one of these patterns points to an unsolved problem. The group itself is accepted as container according to this model. In order to regain the ability to work, the group has to work through and overcome the corresponding basic assumption or conflict pattern.
- The model of group analysis according to Foulkes, whose most important assumption is the existence of an internalised group matrix (1975). This contains the important earlier and currently internalised *object relations* of the group members so that intersubjective

relation patterns but also institutionally formed interaction patterns can be recognised in a group through verbalisation, interaction, or enactment.

Bearing these different supervisory processes in mind, there are three levels of data and information to be gathered in psychoanalytic supervision:

- On the primary level is data on the case in hand: a case can be an individual patient or client but also a group or organisation. The data covers the reason for work with this case and all other information already given. Enactive information also counts as data.
- On the secondary level is the experience of the supervisee—that is, the psychoanalytic social worker, psychoanalyst, teacher, or other participant in the supervision—in the working situation depicted, including this person's *countertransference* in work with his case.
- On the tertiary level is the *transference/countertransference* relationship between the supervisor and supervisee and also the scenic elements as they occur in the supervisory situation.

It is through taking into consideration the *countertransference* and the scenic/enactive elements in the supervisory situation that the *unconscious* or latent communications and meanings are registered (in organisations it would seem to make sense to speak of a latent rather than an *unconscious* sociality, that is, their tendency to set up informal relationships, communications, and also a tendency to form coalitions; see Hondrich, 1997).

*Example case*

In an institution which worked with severely mentally-emotionally disturbed adolescents there was the case of a female member of staff who was threatened and temporarily locked up in a room by a resident when she was on duty alone. She had been able to get out and inform a colleague.

She had in fact been able to get help and so had mastered the situation but had been as if in a state of shock and for a while unable to work. She had not felt sufficiently understood or supported when the situation was talked over and comments had been made by the management of the institution, such as: "In work with adolescents of this kind such things can always happen and one should not overrate their importance."

There had also been a sense of disquiet among the other members of staff in this section so that questions about its continued existence were being raised. In a supervision in which staff and management of the institution took part the effects of this incident and the question of how to proceed were to be resolved.

In the supervision session the member of staff who had been threatened by the young person sat silently, looking rather anxious and scared. One of the managers spoke for her and described with emotion the effect the adolescent's attack had had on her and the staff. The supervisor sensed two concerns here, one emanating from the staff member who had been attacked and the other from the management. The member of staff communicated quite clearly her helplessness and weakness as well as the wish to regain a sense of security, at the same time wordlessly expressing disappointment and something like an atmosphere of reproach towards the management.

On the management side, considerable insecurity and an unspoken sense of guilt were perceptible, covered by a show of understanding and support for her. The supervisor felt a clear appeal from the management to restore good relations with the staff after this upset. What became apparent through enactment rather than words were helplessness, weakness, and reproach on the one side and insecurity, feelings of guilt, and desire to make amends on the other.

In the supervisor's *countertransference* from the member of staff there came an unspoken appeal to "give me protection and security" and from the management an atmosphere oscillating between insecurity, edginess, tension, pressure, and a sense of guilt.

The scene in which the woman had been overpowered was re-created in the supervisory situation with the anxiously silent member of staff overwhelmed by the talking, tense manager, accompanied by the *countertransference* feelings of the supervisor, namely anxiety, a sense of being overwhelmed, and feelings of helpless rage. In this way it became possible to name and work on the real, underlying conflict.

## Supervision in psychoanalytic social work

Psychoanalytic social work is unthinkable without supervision. Psychoanalytic social work is not carried out in a special setting that fosters reflection, as is customary in psychoanalytic treatment, but primarily in the thick of everyday life and practice. The clients of psychoanalytic social work are most of them people suffering from severe mental and emotional conditions such as near psychosis and psychotic, narcissistic, or traumatic illnesses and disorders.

What is common to these illnesses is that they are to a great extent accompanied by processes of *splitting* and externalisation. This is why re-enactments of inner states of emotion occur in current social relationships and this in its turn means that psychoanalytic social workers are always in danger of behaving in accordance with the modes of behaviour of the client's inner *objects* and thus of becoming involved in a repetition of possibly malign intersubjective processes. If this is not recognised, team members will unconsciously take over various different roles of the clients' inner objects and fight out these clients' inner conflicts in the external field.

The instances of team *splitting* that take place in psychiatric institutions are a well-known example of this. They provide evidence of the *unconscious* identifications with the inner objects of the patients (see Becker, 1995b). Supervision in analytic social work can therefore not remain limited to the special case in which something has gone wrong but must take place as a regular, frequent, and continuous accompaniment to work. Supervision not only creates a reflective distance between carer and client which can prevent them from being caught up in destructive acting-out with one another. If this has already happened supervision is there to understand and overcome this pattern. But, beyond this, it creates a sophisticated analysis of relationships with the help of which a client can be better understood in all his social relationships (Gunter, 1994).

If supervision is to be helpful the prerequisites are that the psychoanalytic social workers are willing to take part in it and that the supervisor focusses his interpretation on the patient or client, not on the psychoanalytic social worker (Möller, 2001, p. 49; Pollack, 1995). Further, an atmosphere is required in which, just as in a psychoanalytic treatment, whatever is brought up is taken in and treated as important. Critical judgments make it harder for the supervisee to come out with the things he himself is dissatisfied with or for which he even judges himself harshly. But especially these parts of his work are best suited to point to hidden problems and conflicts. There must therefore be a constructive, accepting, and free atmosphere in supervision in which mistakes and failures are seen as particularly valuable because particularly illuminating.

An example of the supervision of an outpatient institution with the task of caring for HIV-infected patients shows the complicated dynamics which can be produced spontaneously in work with severely disturbed clients.

A social worker and an African working in the same institution are called over to the outpatient section of a hospital which runs an HIV-focus ward.

> In the waiting room they encounter Josie, an African who has been living for about ten years in Germany. She seems anxious and scared. The doctor in charge begins talking to her with a list of questions on her illnesses and living circumstances. He comes across as unfriendly and edgy and talks down to her. The African man translates questions and answers. The social worker gains the impression the woman is preoccupied with something different from the questions she is being asked by the doctor. When asked what she is thinking about she says she is thinking that she doesn't want to live any longer.
>
> The doctor shows no reaction to this information. He simply goes on asking his questions. The woman has been receiving no treatment. She is living with a ten-year-old son. She complains of great weakness, headaches, stomach aches, and aches all over her body. When she stands up it is clear that she is suffering from a one-sided partial paralysis of arm and leg. The doctor is about to discharge her home and hand her over to the care of counselling services. The social worker is horrified, refuses to carry out the discharge, and insists on having her admitted to hospital. She is admitted and on examination she is found, alongside the HIV infection, to have toxoplasmosis and further opportunistic infections, the MRI showing various cerebral defects and oedemata. After three days the woman is discharged.
>
> In the next ten days, when she is repeatedly referred to hospital, further instances of contemptuous, rejecting, and cynical behaviour from the hospital staff occur. In supervision the social worker is indignant, bewildered, and doesn't know what to do about the way the hospital staff are behaving. She considers an official complaint and cannot at the moment imagine how to go on working there.
>
> It is clear that the African patient is in an advanced stage of a so-far untreated HIV infection which is complicated by neurological

symptoms, additional infections, and a re-erupting toxoplasmosis. She needs treatment which can only be given as inpatient treatment. For the staff of the social counselling office it is impossible to understand the irritable, contemptuous, discriminatory, and neglectful behaviour of the hospital staff.

With the help of the African member of staff, to whom the woman has told a good deal, two important pieces of information emerge: she has experienced maltreatment and abuse and the idea of going into hospital puts the fear of death into her. This fear stems from the fact that in her country of origin people only go into hospital when they are terminally ill. She has told him that she is afraid of being killed because people do not want her in Germany.

Now it becomes clear that with her history of maltreatment and abuse she has formed destructive introjects by which she feels threatened with death and this is exacerbated by her belief that hospitals are only for the dying. In this way she has developed the conviction that she is going to be killed and, driven by this conviction she tries to get away from hospital, but on the other hand she shows the staff there a wordless mixture of fatalistic subjection, expectation of maltreatment, fear, anger, hatred, and despair.

With this behaviour she induces in various hospital staff members, particularly in those to whom she ascribes the intention of killing her, a rejecting, irritable, and cynical attitude which is in accordance with her evil, destructive, internalised object representations and with the corresponding conviction that she only deserves bad treatment or even death.

Presumably the fact that the HIV infection had been left untreated was connected with this combination. With the understanding gained in supervision the social worker was able to bring about a change in the attitude of the hospital staff that made cooperation possible and to find a possibility of treatment for the African woman.

Also in cases between institutions and between diverging internal structures inside an institution, psychoanalytic supervision in psychoanalytic social work can provide the decisive contribution to understanding and resolving processes of *splitting* as the expression of inner processes in clients (see also Chapter Eleven). In this way it supports the establishment of a *holding environment* (Winnicott, 1960) such as is often absolutely essential for clients if they are to reach a state of social and mental-emotional stability. As depicted above, supervision at the same time acts as a container for the unprocessed depressive fears and sense of persecution on the part of psychoanalytic social workers which are induced in them by the clients via *projective identification*.

This goal can only be achieved if the work in the supervision session supports stable identification with social work and educational activity and does not try to work towards a "therapeutification" of psychoanalytic social work (Gunter, 1994). There is a danger of this particularly in a field of psychoanalytically orientated social work. The tendency—if it becomes visible—can also be made the subject of supervision, because it, too, has its *unconscious* meaning. It is not something the client can understand if the psychoanalytic social worker bluntly confronts him with an interpretation on the basis of her understanding of the *unconscious* meaning of some piece of behaviour. By contrast as a rule it helps, lightens the burden of difficulties, and fosters change if the social worker can place her extended understanding at the disposal of the client. This is best done by staying as even-tempered as possible in moments of a client's outbreak, refraining from judgmental or punitive comments, and talking over the situation together later to try to understand what has happened so that he can gain new insights and take them on board in the way he behaves. The social worker often needs supervision in order to reach an understanding of the *scene*.

In this way supervision helps the social worker—also in already entangled situations—to gain and repeatedly regain the stance needed to orientate his or her educational and social work activity to a psychodynamic view of psychic and interpersonal processes. The contribution of such supervision supports a relationship-orientated form of social work of great value.

## CHAPTER FOURTEEN

# Quality and qualifications

The descriptions in the previous chapters have shown that psychoanalytic social work is an activity requiring qualified staff, and also that the quality of work has to be ensured through the social worker's constant reflection on his or her own actions.

## *Personal prerequisites*

In many professions the applicants have to fulfil specific preconditions. In some these are clear, particularly if it is a question of the application of technical-instrumental skills. A person wishing to be a dentist or surgeon must have a certain manual deftness and a capacity to think in three dimensions, and no one who suffers from vertigo and a fear of heights should try to take up roof tiling.

In social work, and in particular in psychoanalytic social work, it is far less clear what abilities a social worker should have from the start and what skills he or she can acquire in the course of his work. The case is similar for psychotherapists and psychoanalysts—it is above all a question of psychological abilities and qualities.

This means that personal suitability for the work is crucial. Important elements in this suitability are the capacity for empathy, the ability to practise introspection and self-reflection, and to switch from an experiencing to a reflecting attitude, from a centric to an excentric position.

The psychoanalytic social worker exercises his profession mainly through contacts and encounters which are interwoven with the client's everyday life. This means that he has to allow himself to be involved at close quarters in a relationship with his client and that this relationship is not prestructured or limited as it usually is in a therapeutic arrangement. The result is an "unprotected" face-to-face confrontation with the client's behaviour, his demands, and affects.

Since it is often a question of clients who have a pronounced ability to draw people they meet into entanglements and to induce powerful affects in them, the psychoanalytic social worker has to be aware of the developing tensions and affects to prevent being sucked into them.

Frequently it is not immediately possible to understand what is going on at a particular moment. This requires the ability on the part of the social worker to tolerate not-knowing and not-yet-understanding. At the same time the clients with their frequently severe impairments in the ability to set up contacts and relationships need not only the activity of the social worker to create such contacts but also his sensitivity to the fact that they may wish to be left in peace at a particular moment.

The psychoanalytic social worker therefore needs above all to enjoy being with people and be willing to spend time with interesting, unusual, needy, often exhausting, and even provocative people. He or she must have a sensitivity in making contact with others and be sufficiently curious to understand interactions in order to think over them afterwards either alone or with others.

## Prerequisites—formal basic qualifications

The view of psychoanalytic social work subscribed to in this book, namely the combination of social and instrumental aid with psychoanalytic reflection (see Chapter One), will make it clear that psychoanalytic social work cannot be tied to one single or to just a few related professions. Psychoanalytic social work is a qualified activity or function and not a profession based on a defined education or training.

Nevertheless certain professions are particularly suited as a basic qualification for psychoanalytic social work and are already particularly strongly represented in the field. These are the professions of social pedagogue, social worker, educator, teacher, and psychologist. Alongside these are also professions as yet hardly represented in the field such as educator or preschool teacher, occupational therapist, remedial teacher, and similar occupations. Less frequently to be found in psychoanalytic social work are physicians and nurses from the psychosocial area such as the socio-psychiatric services.

There are craftsmen in vocational education and business studies graduates in psychosocial institutions who may also carry out psychoanalytic social work but they are also rare. A new, certainly very useful basic training for the area of psychoanalytic social work, though not as yet represented in the field, is health science.

As a rule it makes sense to take a degree course, usually in one of the disciplines mentioned: from the point of view of the content this is because psychoanalytic social work is a complex activity which involves a great deal of social interaction and communication, counselling, systemic thinking, planning, and self-reflection; and then from the pragmatic point of view, because social status is to a large extent connected with formal qualifications. If psychoanalytic social workers have good formal qualifications it increases their chances of gaining recognition: they gain more attention and remuneration, and they have improved chances of being able to carry through new treatment and approaches to care and also of acquiring funding for projects.

### Extending competence—self-awareness, continuing development, and further training

The professions mentioned above form the basis for further qualifications which aid psychoanalytic social work. Since work with the client is a central element in psychoanalytic social work and because in this work attentive awareness of self is indispensable, it is eminently helpful to carry out an extensive training in self-awareness. This also helps one to become more aware of one's own prejudices, fears, and blind spots.

Above all it creates an experience of the effects of *transference* with which every member of staff in psychoanalytic social work is constantly confronted in working with clients. The staff learn to recognise their individual response to the *transferences* they are presented with, that is, their own *countertransference* and relate this to their clients. This part of self-awareness is one that a beginner can best acquire through a personal analysis.

146    PSYCHOANALYTIC SOCIAL WORK

There is a further part of self-knowledge that can best be gained in an encounter group. This is the experience of how one behaves spontaneously in social encounters, what goes on inside one, and what effect one has on a partner in interaction. The experience of self in group encounter is particularly helpful for psychoanalytic social work because psychoanalytic social work does not take place in a special situation apart, but rather in everyday encounters and interactions which are very little regulated. In these situations attentive introspection is less important than intuitive action and response in a contact.

The extent of self-exploration undertaken is something to be decided individually. It depends on an individual's personality and his or her previous experiences with self-awareness. As regards the experience of group encounters, as well as a continuous participation in a group, it makes sense to have experience in a group setting over several days—a "group laboratory". It is in the density of this longer period of being in a group that regressive dynamics emerge more clearly, and these are what occur in the general living areas of institutions where staff and residents keep meeting and where they spend a lot of time together.

As in every profession, continuous development makes excellent sense. It can be in the form of case-based supervision or it can be orientated towards a particular method or theory. Appropriate locations today for such further training, beyond the confines of the institution where one is working, are conferences for psychoanalytic social work, courses for training in psychoanalytic psychosis therapy, programmes for psychoanalytic teaching, single events in psychoanalytic training institutes, for example those concerned with psychoanalytic developmental theory or psychoanalytic social and cultural theory, and a number of training courses in the area of social work. Courses of this kind are offered at the present time in a number of psychoanalytic institutes and some psychiatric hospitals which are open to psychoanalytic thinking and in the Uk also in conferences and seminars organized by the International Association of Forensic Psychotherapy (IAFP).

Systematic extension of competence that leads to work at a higher quality grade in a section of the profession is as a rule recognised as professional development. In this sense psychoanalytic social work itself can be regarded as the acquisition of further competence for various basic professions. It is not as yet organised in this form. Various further training courses are, however, very useful for psychoanalytic social work, even if they come under different headings and are only open to certain professions. For instance, there are courses for further education in psychoanalysis for medical doctors and psychologists at the psychoanalytic institutes of the scientific psychoanalytical associations. There is also the further training to become an analytic child and adolescent psychotherapist which is offered to social pedagogues, social workers, and teachers, in addition to the professions mentioned before, again at psychoanalytic institutes.

## On a form of further professional development in psychoanalytic social work

Up to now no systematic and formalised further training in psychoanalytic social work has been set up. The wide variety of possible principal professions and the basic courses in psychoanalytic social work offered to those in them demonstrates that there is as yet no systematised or organised approach. Since the area which could benefit from psychoanalytic social work is very wide one would expect to find interest in continuous development among many in the social field. Working out a curriculum and disseminating it in a course would enable targeted consideration of the needs of the most important fields of practice.

A possible curriculum should cover

– a theoretical part with psychoanalytic developmental theory, theory of the *unconscious*, general psychoanalytic nosology, psychoanalytic theory of society and culture, psychoanalytic group theory, psychoanalytic theory of institutions, psychoanalytic interaction theory, foundations of psychoanalytic theory of education;
– a practical part with work experience in an institution working according to the principles of psychoanalytic social work, participation in supervision groups and mediation processes;

a part concerned with the development of self-awareness in a one-to-one setting and in a group setting.

Further training and education can be offered in two forms, one for young people just starting work, which would consist of a full-day course to be held at a university or polytechnic, organised as a master's course with access for graduates in social work, sociology, theory of education, and psychology, and another set up for those with several years' experience of work in the social field. Both forms should be courses leading to a state-recognised degree. Courses of this kind could be offered by an independent body but that would require considerable preparatory work to achieve the necessary recognition and status.

## Good everyday work—discussion of cases, case-, team-, and institutional supervision

Psychoanalytic social work requires the frequent creation of space for reflection. The reflective space enables distancing from the interactions with clients and thus observation of them from outside the situation which is necessary to clarify the social worker's own contribution. This excentric position is achieved in the triangulated setting of supervision. In supervision the *position of the third* is created by the setting, which is apart from everyday work, and by the supervisor (cf. Chapter Thirteen). Alongside working for understanding through reflection, supervision also acts as a container for the hard-to-bear, not-yet-understood happenings that are part of social work and thus has a function in alleviating affective stress.

Supervision can focus on various levels in an institution. Experience shows that supervisions carried out over a longer period of time tend to cover all levels—case, team, institution—since they are interconnected and influence one another. The case-based supervision is at the same time an important element in further internal training. In the careful group contemplation of all the information on one client, a paradigmatic understanding is created every time and continues to have an effect on two levels. On one level a method for the contemplation of a case and for its interpretation is practised, and this over time becomes internalised and is available for later cases. At the same time on another level the individual client becomes an internalised representation of a particular arrangement of conflicts and problems. He becomes a building block of experiential knowledge which is indispensable for good work.

In team supervision, conflicts which had not till then been visible in case-centred supervision can come to light in the form of mirroring. The reason for this lies in the susceptibility of groups, also of a team, to regressive processes so that in a group deeper layers of the *unconscious* present themselves in *scenic or enactive* form. Many conflicts that occur in a team can then be understood as mirrorings of work with the clients and unresolved conflicts there. A different kind of conflict is one with its roots in the team itself, which is not to be understood as the mirroring of work with clients. The resolution of these conflicts in supervision is equally important as they can impair or destroy the ability of the team to do their work. It is also important to examine whether such unresolved conflicts have affected work with the clients.

Institutional supervision observes the processes in an institution and the atmosphere to which the management makes a significant contribution. The institutional processes and the atmosphere are of great importance because the institution as a whole is experienced by the staff as a *maternal container* which—when it is positive—holds, nourishes, rewards, and shows understanding. When it is negative, the container does not fulfil these functions and conveys to the staff a feeling of homelessness and disorganisation.

A stressful institutional atmosphere makes itself felt in the frequent mention of institutional and management issues in case and team supervisions. After a certain period if institutional conflicts remain unresolved it is usually the case that the sick rate of an institution rises.

A further problem which can only be resolved by including the institutional level is the development of an institutional *defence* against the real task of the institution. The *defence* against forming relationships with the client in social psychiatry (Bruns, 1998) can be regarded as an example of this.

The therapeutic chain was developed in social psychiatry in the 1980s. Its fundamental principle was always to pass on patients or clients from one section to the next after a certain time when they began to improve. Through this process the relationships which had just been built up were broken off and the patient had to start all over again building up new ones in the new place. The central element in psychotherapy, according to all research results, is, however, precisely the therapeutic relationship. Improvements in the condition of the patient are normally related to the fact that a patient has developed trust and this means that he or she has set up a relationship.

But to allow the member of staff conducting the therapy to get involved in a relationship confronts him or her with unprocessed inner conflicts and with the internalised, often bleak, and dismal relationship representations of the client, which reappear when a serious therapeutic relationship is established in the *transference/countertransference* relationship. To avoid this experience the establishment of a relationship is warded off.

The organisation of custodial psychiatry (with all the overtones of the word custodial in this classic term) but also of social psychiatry amounted to, or indeed still amounts to, the avoidance of a therapeutic relationship in which these pathologically significant and internalised relationships could be worked on. It is a case of the institutional warding off of an effective therapeutic relationship.

Also important for day-to-day work—but to be distinguished from supervision—is case discussion. In this setting, information about a client which staff need to know is passed on, plans are created for a client's development and their implementation is checked. Case discussions are held with the circle of members of staff and serve to ensure that all the staff have all the important, current information about a client. They also make sure the goals for one client do not go in different directions and prevent the staff from being played off against each other by the clients.

Just like any individual, all institutions also need regular self-reflection. It serves to check whether they are still pursuing the goals they have set themselves or whether they have at any point been distracted from them. It is in the peculiar nature of institutions to evolve their own dynamics stemming from the external social interactions in which they are involved and from their inner-institutional dynamics. These dynamics can lead institutions in a direction which is different from the one they were designed for. Since institutions in a sense "take over" the people working for them, they are more powerful than their staff and appear as the representatives of a social contract or law. Individual members of an institution, even if they are in leading managerial positions, will most often not be able to reflect on the institution, its aims, and its task with any critical distance.

The task of an institution is usually determined by what it has done in the past. This is the source of its overwhelming tendency to persist as it is and its justification for continuing in the future. Thus, essentially, the institution relies on its existence in the past. One good opportunity to reflect on the activities, tasks, and goals of an institution and to detect possible discrepancies between aims and actual practice are conferences and research activities. At conferences it is possible to present one's own activities, open them to discussion, and check whether these activities really make sense and are necessary. This process yields particularly good results if the work processes in an institution and their results are accompanied by research activities in the widest sense. Research demands that one refrain from naively losing oneself in institutional processes. Instead one has to evaluate them from a distance and question how much sense they make. In this respect research and its presentation at conferences open to the scholarly community in the field can be regarded as a systematised self-reflection analogous to supervision. It helps to prevent an institution from regarding self-preservation as its central task. Such research and public presentation of a person's own work at conferences can be beneficial in yet another way: in the course of working on the lectures those involved have to reflect deeply about their work, and for them particularly this effort creates what is probably the most fruitful form of professional development imaginable.

## CHAPTER FIFTEEN

# Psychoanalytic social work in practice at the Verein für Psychoanalytische Sozialarbeit Rottenburg/Tübingen

## Teaching and learning from experience

Over the last thirty years the staff of the Verein für Psychoanalytische Sozialarbeit Rottenburg/Tübingen have been developing concepts for psychoanalytic social work in inpatient, partly inpatient, and outpatient form.

For the history and structure of the Verein and its units—outpatients, into-work project, therapeutic home, see Allerdings and Staigle (1999) and the web site at www.psychoanalytische-sozialarbeit-tue.de.

The inpatient and outpatient services of the Verein für Psychoanalytische Sozialarbeit began their work with just a few adolescents suffering from severe psychiatric disorders with autistic and psychotic symptoms. In the course of time the number of clients has grown and the spectrum of their disorders broadened considerably.

However, the shared invention of appropriate setting constructions is a complex and slow process particularly when an institution is first establishing itself. It develops in work with people who suffer from mental-emotional disorders more easily than with those with antisocial disorders because their acting-out is slower and allows one more time and space to think.

Perhaps this is one reason why a number of attempts to set up institutions of psychoanalytic social work, which started for historical or present-day reasons in other fields of work (i.e., work with families or with antisocial adolescents), had a harder time developing stable concepts and setting constructions.

How can one conceptualise psychoanalytic social work? Psychoanalytic social work unites aspects of all three "impossible professions"— psychoanalysis, education, and government—of which Sigmund Freud wrote (1937c).

These three professions—impossible in the sense that it is impossible to create operational definitions for them—are anyway excluded in the traditional view: for an ideal "pure" psychoanalysis, for instance, it is regarded as essential to abstain consistently from all actions connected with governing or educating, that is, all actions that directly intervene in the internal but even more in the external life circumstances of the analysand.

But if psychoanalysis wishes to encounter and help people whose psychic structure expresses itself not only in intrapsychic but also primarily in interpersonal conflict, it seems one is compelled to turn to the register of educative measures and ways of managing the environment—"governing" action, and therefore has to give up the position of abstinence. In psychoanalytic social work we seek ways of making moments of governing, educating, and analysing interact beneficially in a reflected fashion.

We do this together with young people whose life difficulties place them somewhere in the overlapping areas of psychiatry, education, social work in youth services, aid for the disabled, and analytic psychotherapy. They need a particular form of help such as psychoanalytic social work can offer. This is characterised by being flexibly adapted to the mental-emotional structures and social problems of its clients— and not the other way round, where clients have to adapt to the given structures of an institution and institutional programmes.

In concrete terms this means in our Verein twenty-five full-time employees and ten supervisors work together to achieve this individual fit for the help offered and its constructive effectiveness, using the minimum of means. This staff provides responsible, judicially accountable outpatient support for around sixty people and part-residential for a dozen.

The following contributions illustrate some spectra of our work in examples. In this description we centre on Max, Michael, Miriam,

Gustav, Werner, and Jonas, taking as a starting point the individual previous history and problems of these children, adolescents, young adults, adults, and their parents, and depicting here our attempts to construct a setting and a helpful mode of dealing with each of them geared to their specific problems in life.

In doing so we have placed the emphasis on either the concrete (social work) establishment of the external framework and setting or on the (therapeutic) inner processes of encounters, and describe these in excerpts from outpatient and inpatient work. Martin Feuling outlines psychoanalytic social work as the attempt to give impulses to the development of inner spaces and structures using constructions of concrete external spaces where, as in the examples of Max and Michael, these intrapsychically operant structures have been insufficiently developed.

Also in the outpatient field of the Verein, Joachim Staigle depicts sections of his work with an autistic-psychotic boy, Werner. Sylvia Künstler describes how setting constructions need to be adjusted to the client's life situations as they vary in the case of care for a young woman. From the Hagenwört group home for young adults Horst Nonnenmann offers us insight into inpatient work, and Olaf Schmidt from the Therapeutic Home for Children and Adolescents reports on work with Jonas.

## On the link between inner and outer

One of our fundamental working hypotheses is that in psychoanalytic social work intrapsychic spaces that have not been developed first of all have to be "constructed" as concrete external spaces (cf. Verein für Psychoanalytische Sozialarbeit, 1993). We use the term "construction" in the sense of Freud's concept of "constructions in analysis" (1937d).

A relationship structure has to be created for clients in their tangible external social reality until the external places become internalised, contribute to complementing the psychic agencies, and can finally be symbolised. All in- and outpatient settings are built on the following frame of four different places, forms of encounter, living spaces, forms of discourse:

1. The place for living and surviving, not greatly structured in terms of time and content: everyday life, provision, and subsistence
2. The place for learning and working, clearly structured for time and content

3. The place for analytical individual sessions, structured clearly for time but not for content and which are at the centre of every setting
4. The hardly comprehensible, complex places of mystery in the social sphere outside our setting.

In each individual case we work on setting up the relation between these four places in a way that the client and the people around him can live in them and in a way that will enable the client's development. Our principle here is to place as little as possible within the four walls of our institution and rather to try to involve as many other institutions as possible in establishing a setting: as a result the cooperation with other institutions makes up a large part of our work.

## Max A

Max (cf. Feuling, 1997) was referred to us with the psychiatric diagnosis of Asperger's syndrome. He had shown signs of it early on with autistoid behaviour patterns but had been able to stay in the normal school system until the beginning of puberty. From then on the school was unable to handle him as he did not respect any boundaries whatever. Inpatient treatment was not considered because his mentally-emotionally disordered parents were against it and he sided with them.

Attempts to keep him in individual schooling at the school which was incorporated in the child and adolescent psychiatric clinic of his home town failed on the grounds of his externalising and antisocial behaviour.

Engaging a social pedagogic family help was tried at his home but also failed as she was unable to set up a helpful milieu for Max's development there. Finally, with nothing to hold onto, Max spent his time riding around alone on trams and telephoning everyone he had ever had contact with and whose phone number he could remember. An inpatient psychotherapy was impossible to set up because his parents saw no need for it and were not under sufficient psychological stress to seek help. All educational outpatient approaches had failed.

As there was no help to be had in the major town forty kilometres away, at the age of fifteen and for the following six years he landed at the Verein: five days a week he set off early on a one-and-a-half-hour journey by bus and train, travelling back home again in the evening, and in this way spent six to eight hours there.

The staff established the setting which was designed and modified for him for three of the above named places in the following manner:

**The place for living and surviving**: At first, staff went out with Max to lunch at a pub; this soon became intolerable and they began to provide lunch in the waiting room of the Verein for him and increasingly for other youngsters. These mealtime situations were handled by all the members of staff in turn with no specifically designated person for him alone. The waiting room developed over three to four years into a supportive place in which he could feel safe without being looked after and he was able to keep to minimal social rules. By playing on the computer or writing he was able to handle times of being alone there and even made contact with other youngsters. As time went on the day he spent at the Verein was reduced after his integration into working life had progressed enough for him to have his midday meal at the workshop.

**The place of learning and working**: In the first year Max was given first one and then two daily lessons on his own at the Verein; in the second and third year he went to the clinic school in a very small group for up to three hours daily, an arrangement which functioned—in contrast to what had happened in his home town—because we kept a member of staff on call for the school to turn to at any time for support if he broke the rules. Max was not able, however, to achieve a school qualification of any kind because of his autistoid *defence* against learning anything new. In the fourth year Max made his first attempts at working in our house, with increasing contacts with a workshop for mentally and emotionally disturbed people. Gradually he was able to cope with being at the workshop for longer periods of time, a phase which was accompanied by regular mediating and counselling talks between one of our staff and the staff at the workshop. Step by step his working hours were extended to cover a full working day.

**The place of individual analytic sessions**: I am not going to describe in detail what developed in these individual sessions since I wish to focus here above all on the external construction of the setting (cf. Feuling, 1997).

In general one can say that within the framework of the individual sessions there is room for anything that is on an adolescent's mind so long as it doesn't break the mould. At the outset of work with an adolescent the individual analytic sessions are one part of the whole setting which is primarily characterised by being totally different from the other parts and places and should be determined as little as possible by therapeutic goals. The more disturbed a person is in his psychic and social functions the more sensitively he is aware of the uniqueness of the analytic space which can emerge in these individual sessions. The concrete shape of the individual sessions develops in this shared work out of the recognition that the client experiences (cf. Verein für Psychoanalytische Sozialarbeit, 1997).

In the beginning Max had four hours a week with a female member of staff. This soon proved too constricting, hurtful, and taxing for both of them so that on two days a male analytic therapist joined them, intended as a fatherly, protective, and boundary-setting figure, a concrete third person, in view of Max's tendency, in his maternal *transference*, to attack and overstep the boundaries of what was bearable for the female staff member.

The now-present, now-absent function of the additional therapist as third person was, however, so little internalised by Max and so little effective when the therapist was *not* there that the member of staff was only able to keep up the individual sessions over three years in the presence or with the on-call availability of a male third person. She finally finished her work with Max after four years because the actual presence of the third person became indispensable and the male therapist took over her place. Towards the end of Max's time he had two individual sessions a week with him.

**Places of mystery**: The long journeys with the variety of social contacts involved were fundamentally outside our sphere of influence. With his increasing development, Max's radius of movement increased in Tübingen, the place of therapy, and in his home town. He showed more and more independent activity.

After his time with us was over Max worked in his home town for forty hours a week in a sheltered workshop for mentally and emotionally disordered people and went once a week to a local therapist. He remained living with his parents.

## Michael B

Michael (cf. Bosch & Feuling, 1997) came to us with the psychiatric diagnosis of borderline syndrome. He was suffering from marked fears. From earliest childhood on he had been conspicuous for aggressive and destructive actions directed against objects and people. At the age of ten he was placed in a boys' home with a psychoanalytic working concept. There he carried out a number of aggressive attacks on boys and adults, but also suffered such attacks himself.

For half a year he was placed in a secure adolescent unit. There the situation escalated in alternating perpetrator and victim roles. A further group home found they could not keep him after half a year. Michael, by this time fourteen years old, was admitted to an adolescent psychiatric hospital. After nine months this institution reached the limits of its ability to tolerate his behaviour and discharged him, first of all to a guest house.

Since the framework of a group did not seem conceivable, a single room flat was set up for the now just fifteen-year-old with individual social pedagogic care and, parallel to that, individual sessions with a therapist in the adolescent psychiatric unit.

This attempt, too, failed after a short time because it was soon beyond the scope of educational approaches to find responses to the psychotic parts of his behaviour. Michael himself found a foster family which took him in for a few further months until the incident when he broke a glass bottle over the au pair's head. After six months in two psychiatric clinics he was referred to the Verein. He was sixteen when he arrived. He is now over thirty and care for him is still needed and provided.

He managed to wear down our framework very close to the limits of our endurance. Looking back we now think that in the early phases we were not able to pick up and respond to his very complex psychic structure, characterised by *splitting* processes. This structure contained layers of autistoid-schizophrenic, neurotic, and above all paranoid forms of *defence*. Particularly the perception and consideration of the paranoid aspects in creating a setting for him was what made our work with him over many years possible.

The setting invented for him developed in the following manner. Originally three colleagues started on the work with Michael. This number, however, soon had to be raised to five, mainly because we could not otherwise have covered for absences through holidays and sick leave since Michael was not able to go more than two, or at most three days without contact with us. Currently he still has four carers. A centring of the analytic function on one person is soon to be implemented. He has two contact sessions of an hour per day with his carers but stays in the house at times for a number of hours: he seeks protection from the loneliness of his flat that makes him depressive and the paranoid-schizoid *defence* against this depression which takes the form of destructive, aggressive acting-out in social relations.

In the course of his development Michael exerted a marked influence on the form of encounter that his carers offered. Our experience with him as with others is that the person who is defined at the outset as the analyst is avoided and that instead the person who first takes over practical, everyday, and provisioning functions is shifted into the analytical position. Then the social worker does not avoid the analytic position and refer his client to the analyst, but seeks instead to take over the analytic position himself (cf. on this point Freud, 1925f).

**The place for the everyday and survival**: At the start of our work Michael made it clear what he felt he needed: a carer he could call on at any time but that he could also send away at any time. We countered this wish to be omnipotent with an offer of defined and limited contact times which he constantly tried to extend during his times spent in the house.

It was soon clear that Michael needed little concrete support in the area of practical life skills and that, on the contrary, offers of help in this area were quickly felt by him to be persecutory because they touched on his dependency. The nurturing aspect took the form of sharing meals with him alone or in a small group and this, with his unaccompanied periods spent in the waiting room, represented his everyday pattern in the total setting.

**The place of learning and working**: A first attempt at working in a self-help company (electro recycling) soon failed as a result of aggressive collisions with colleagues. Since then he had gone over to the workshop twice a week and carried material home to work on there for about two hours a day. He had again and again been close to breaking off this job in protest against the lonely character of the work and the dependency he experienced in it.

**The place of individual analytic sessions**: Michael needed three of his four carers to be the particular recipients of his split *transferences*, which were gathered together in a weekly supervision to be reflected on. Perhaps one could say—to exaggerate a little—that it was above all in this supervision circle that the analytic space developed. The more dominant the paranoid fears are in a case the more important it is that the supervision setting is transparent for the client. In clients with a more neurotic structure the question arises as to whether the therapist of the individual sessions should take part at all in the supervision of the multi-person setting and, if so, how much he should tell the carers who are in other functions.

**The place of mystery**: Of the 168 hours in a week Michael spent twenty to thirty in our house, the rest of the time he structured for himself: he had a variety of contacts which he was, however, easily liable to destroy with his psychotic acting-out, though he was able to keep some of them for longer periods. Distrustful as he was, he reacted sensitively and allergically to institutions with their tendency to have an institutionalised controlling, persecuting, and forbidding *countertransference*. Michael had been, for example, attached to a psychiatric institution, where he was seen by a series of doctors in the outpatient clinic over a number of years, but which all of a sudden refused him further outpatient psychiatric treatment despite his still continuing severe disorder.

On the whole one can say that we managed to work through the predominance of his paranoid-schizoid *defence* mechanisms (they are characterised by *splitting* and projective mechanisms which "remove" the "bad", unwanted parts of a person, projecting them in his *unconscious* conviction into another person), to the point where Michael today more often shows the more integrated state of the *depressive position* (i.e., a state of simultaneously integrating and tolerating "good" and "bad", wanted and unwanted aspects of oneself). This is presumably only possible because of the scattered character of our institution, but there was always the danger that the dormant violence in him might erupt and be directed against others or against himself. Because this danger was always present the supervision circle had to deal with many questions over whether we could take the ethical and judicial responsibility for the framework we gave him. Supervision created the psychic space to take in and defuse his destructive impulses.

## Years with Werner

### A brief account of his previous history

I met Werner when he was thirteen years old. He lived with his grandmother in dangerously cramped isolation. Any other spaces where he might have been able to develop outside the family had collapsed. The grandmother refused to let him be looked after as an inpatient in a child and adolescent psychiatric unit. A part of his development was the experience of early deprivation with repeated traumatic loss of the main supportive emotional relationships to maternal-holding persons.

Werner was born as the child of an unmarried mother still living with her mother. Up to the age of two and a half months he lived with his mother who, it seems, rejected him from the start and did not provide for him sufficiently. He had bedsores and was underfed. He cried as well beyond what was normal. The grandmother on the father's side took him in. Because she was out working he was looked after by the great-grandmother, who lived in the house, as did Werner's father, too. The father took no responsibility for his son's financial support; he was only occasionally in work and lived in a state of neglect on the fringes of society. The grandmother was the most important carer and he received various forms of care and treatment because of serious symptoms. The loss of relationships was repeated in premature termination of these treatments.

Werner's aggressive behaviour took a turn for the worse when he was eleven and a half. For instance he began to hit older women with a stick. He is said to have commented they were going to die soon anyway. He also attacked smaller children, hitting, biting, and scratching them. He often ran away and turned up as a tormenting spirit in a kindergarten. He did not seem to be able to feel any fear or sense of remorse. According to a report from the school the difficulties had erupted with this intensity after his grandmother had said Werner was to look after her when he grew up. Finally he was expelled as being impossible to integrate and he received six hours a week schooling at home.

## The first interview

When Werner was introduced to me in our first personal contact I saw an attractive, curly-headed, loose-knit boy facing me. In the presence of a number of people he appeared to be shy, insecure and very "good". He made rather curious, clumsy movements and sudden, uncoordinated gestures. When we withdrew into another room together the situation changed instantly. At first I was astonished that he had a command of such differentiated and expressive language but I hardly had time to adjust to him. He bombarded me immediately with a continuous stream of questions.

"Have you ever cried? When do you cry? I know you. Where do you live? How old are you? What happens if there's a tooting and I am at the door? I want to see your key. Do you have a watch? Was it ever broken? What did you do to it? Why don't you throw it away? Have you got a car? Has it ever broken down? I must check the engine. I'm an electrician, you see."

In between the sentences he made gestures, movements, and noises that sounded like engines. "That's my tractor, it has 100,000 horsepower, perhaps even fifty or thirty. That's my boss sitting in the back. You can't see the tractor and the boss. Do you have spectacles? I must make them squeak, I can make music out of them. That's petrol and off she goes, the old banger!" Alongside his stream of questions and comments he searched around the room and commandeered everything that wasn't nailed down. If anything interested him he tooted as if he had a built-in horn, toot-toot. The room was new to me and he started turning it upside-down. I began to be worried because within moments he had created chaos. Any remark that came from me, if I suggested a game or picked up any interest he showed, was ignored. He seemed to need to dominate the situation completely. I didn't seem to exist as a person for him. He turned me into a marionette through the way he fired questions at me and negated my presence with the way he whirled around the room.

When he came upon a neurological examination instrument I felt called on to intervene and tell him to put things back in order. At that he flashed round towards me with a sharp-pointed pinwheel and ran it over my hand in one rapid movement. "Do you cry when I hurt you?" Suddenly angry, I took the instrument away from him, inwardly shocked at my reaction, and I sensed my fear of getting injured. I told him that I was strong enough to deal with him without getting hurt. "I don't believe that, I'm stronger than you are." When I contradicted him he said: "You only want to kill me but I'm going to shoot myself anyway soon, do away with myself," and at this moment I saw tears come to his eyes and I was aware of a sense of great sadness. When I said to him, "You must be sad," he grew furious and kicked at me. "You arsehole!" Then he played for a while at the washbasin, which seemed to calm him down. Suddenly he wanted to play a game with me. I was to pretend to be asleep. Then he took my watch from my wrist. He tooted to wake me up. Now I was supposed to discover he had stolen my watch and at my pretended shock he burst into uncontrollable laughter. He repeated this a number of times with variations. Most of the time I was now supposed to be a small child that couldn't resist his raids and was very scared of him. Interestingly I found this game with him, in which he was the producer and I was given every line I was allowed to say, far more unpleasant and difficult to bear than his attacks on the furnishings and contents of the room, because I was made downright defenceless and was afraid he could really hurt me when I was pretending to be asleep. I was relieved when Werner and I rejoined the others. Suddenly he was a "good boy" again, asking me if I was going to visit him again soon.

The impression that I had gained in the first meeting mirrored and confirmed my first emotional reaction to the previous history of the child. Werner's central problem, as I saw it, was that he had never in his life experienced a sufficiently secure and nurturing environment. Too early, before he was capable of bearing separations, he repeatedly lost the connection to his most important attachment figure. There was also never a father. The presence of an effective father might have enabled the mother to adapt to the new situation and provide for the child better. Such a father figure might have served as an identification figure and enabled a triangulated solution to emerge from the symbiotic relationship to the mother figure. In the further stages of his life the loss of his most important significant others outside the family was often repeated. Closely connected to the losses were the primitive *defence* mechanisms against psychotic fears and threat of disintegration which manifested in Werner's difficulties. One thread running through the story of his life was the central problem of aggression towards himself and others, a form of *defence* against inner void and lifelessness.

Spontaneously I liked Werner. I could imagine working with him over years. And yet in the encounter what predominated were the elements of destructiveness and unbearableness. This encounter destroyed any previously constructed picture I had of what I might be able to do with him. I was sure then that he would have to remain the one with the greatest say and that I, as his counterpart, would represent hardly more than a puppet or marionette. I experienced him as a burden and a plague. He came intolerably close to me: this showed outwardly in his unceasing questioning to which I was hardly allowed to respond. Pivotal in the treatment would presumably be the question of whether the two of us would emerge from the relationship alive and unscathed or whether we would break off this relationship, too, out of resignation and despair.

## First attempts at understanding and design of settings

I tried to understand the striking aspects of his behaviour. It seemed to me that he had not been able to develop a secure inner attachment to a good inner *object* because his primary carers had not adapted their behaviour to his needs. This meant he had to experience the physical separation from his carer at too early a stage, before he was capable of bearing physical separations and privations. Since at this stage of development self and *object* are not yet separated in the inner world, severe privations—as in the nurture by the carer—take on the quality of the loss of a part of the body. In other words such early traumatic experience leads to fears of loss and of being annihilated. It seems Werner had been unable to bear these fears and this psychic pain and that they threatened his mental and emotional integrity with fears of complete breakdown.

As a small child Werner was not able to form any secure inner representations of holding relationships and is therefore up to the present day dependent on a relationship to an idealised *object*. He depends on having his carers physically present and they must not expect him to cope with privations and separations. In day-to-day living what this meant for Werner was that all experiences of opposition to his immediate impulses, all experiences of separation and confrontations with reality which might diminish the idealisations of the carers he revered, triggered fears for his very existence. These were fears that he absolutely could not bear and he therefore could not consciously sense or symbolise them. The *defence* against these fears was carried out mainly through not being much or at all aware of himself. For his own protection he had to ward off from himself the threatening psychotic fears, revived in real present-day experiences of being deprived of what he needed, with the help of primitive *defence* processes.

He developed *autistic defence* mechanisms and other psychotic processes which, although they were the expression of a failed psychic development, were at the same time the creative and constructive activities of a psyche threatened with total breakdown and were aimed at maintaining the functioning of his psyche even if only in reduced form.

Since separation from our institution would have seemed to both of us like a renewed failure in the setting up of a constructive relationship, his worsened state raised the question of whether a form of outpatient care could be set up which could substitute for the inpatient support or treatment which was in fact needed. In this situation a setting for Werner's care had to take various aspects into account. It had to offer him a high degree of security, constancy, and reliability to avoid break-ing off yet another relationship. In view of his impending puberty and the existing retardation in his development it was a question of plan-ning for care to be available over a span of many years.

Werner needed schooling alongside therapeutic care. The setting for outpatient psychoanalytic socio-therapeutic care that needed to be set up also had to offer Werner and his grandmother a way of structuring everyday life and concrete day-to-day support, for instance by provid-ing meals. The outpatient setting had to substitute for what was not achievable, namely admittance to inpatient treatment. It turned out that with schooling integrated into the therapeutic frame we could provide the *splitting* possibilities needed for this care programme in a multiple-person framework. With social worker and teacher available there were now two people who could separately take on aspects of relationship work that would have clashed. And this meant that via the integration of these different aspects in us, his carers, over time Werner was increas-ingly able to experience himself as a whole person.

### Play sessions with Werner

To give a clearer idea of the protective mechanisms that Werner used and of the structure of the relationship that developed between us, typi-cal aspects of the course of our play sessions together are described in the following.

At the beginning of the session he would go straight to the wall, press on an imaginary button to start the play machine, while saying: "I have got a cassette with me on which today's session is recorded." He seemed to have identified himself with a cassette recorder and with its possibilities of prestructuring and so being able to steer himself and the anxiety-inducing situation of encounter. In certain areas he seemed to identify himself not with people but with far more predictable objects such as cars or electrical apparatus.

After he had "switched on" the game in his own way he became the person who prescribed exactly, with very few exceptions, what I was to do or say and who was on no account going to allow me to act as an independent, feeling, and thinking person. He played through phantasies with me in which it seemed it was *not* a question of phantasies but that what we were playing was a shared reality.

In these games I had to be myself or a person from my personal circle but also other "kids in specs" etc. Werner did not play in any symbolic sense. The situations for which he was "the producer" were real for him. He was then the Werner who terrorised me in a wide variety of ways, tormented me, and placed me in situations of hope followed by the inevitable disappointment of these hopes. For instance he played with me that he was crashing into my home on a mechanical digger. He then tormented or shot my child and my wife before my very eyes. While he was doing this he said, "You should see your face now!" He knew that my daughter had just been born. In the game he ran her over in front of me with his great digger, held her out of the window, or carried her off home to have thousands of kids in specs of his own. Now he began to get closer to me. I was, he said, a small kid in specs and could not defend myself. In a flash he ran over my face with his tongue, wanted to kiss me, snuggle up to me, and also bite and squeeze me. In such moments the slightest sign of resistance from me or the setting up of any rule to protect my physical boundaries unleashed an outbreak of fury and attacks on me in which he tried to bite me, scratch me, but above all spit on me and smear me with snot. If I held him, for his and my protection, he cried out in tears and despair. "I am not going live much longer anyway, I'm going to electrocute myself. I hate you. You don't love me. You hate me, you will be happy when I am dead." If I tried to calm him and comfort him he asked me if I would cry if he died, but added straight away, in a resigned tone, "You'd only pretend to cry, you wouldn't really cry." But it was only through really experiencing and taking in the idea that it was I who was sad and not he himself that he seemed able to calm down.

Over a long period this kind of playing was almost intolerable for me and I could only expose myself to it knowing that it would be over at an appointed time. During the game a murderous hatred of Werner would well up inside me, an immense need not to let myself be ordered around and terrorised. The degree of helplessness and exposure to his attacks felt unbearable to me and led to situations in which I also began to act out. In the course of the game I had begun to reach a state in which I could no longer distinguish between playing and reality. I really felt threatened and exposed to feelings of hatred and fear in identification with the victim position. In some situations I developed an extreme fear of Werner and above all was afraid the next moment he would put my eyes out if I didn't do something that very instant. If, however, I even moved a fraction at such a moment when Werner was standing there threatening me with a screwdriver in his hand he would begin to attack me as if he were threatened by me. At such moments I lost my ability to think so that I could find hardly any way of inwardly distancing myself.

## Where he lived

During the whole of the time he was in our care Werner continued to live with his grandmother. We had a weekly talk with her which served to further understanding, to deal with the frequent crisis situations, and also to exchange reports of what happened from day to day. These talks looked at finding possible ways to set up changes in the way the two of them lived together, particularly to accommodate Werner's clear separation and individuation needs. A separation of Werner from his grandmother in the sense of a concrete separation that would have enabled him to move out and join a group of same-age young people was finally not achievable. There was simply too much mutual mental-emotional and material dependence. Werner reacted to this situation by creating a completely independent area inside the house the two of them shared. Here he had an autonomous area free of the provision and care offered by his grandmother: a small kitchen, his own fridge and his own food. In the garden he put up a little shed with several rooms in it made from odds and ends found at the recycling centre. He called it "my ranch", with a "café" (coffee machine for the visitors he longed for), a "workshop" (hundreds of defunct pieces of apparatus given him or picked up), and a "casino pub" (the one-armed bandit given him by his father). Only the customers were missing. However, after work and at weekends he had something to do here. This was his home—separate from his grandmother's sphere. He also had friends of both sexes, sporadically, most of them as bizarre as himself. And there were always understanding adults who kept in touch with him or were able to stand his contact with them.

Werner is now thirty-seven years old. Every year at Christmas and on his birthday I write him a letter. He rings me up to thank me, and asks how I am and how things are with the people and objects that connect (or separate) us: my children, my wife, my car, the outpatient unit, Elfriede, the teacher. And he asks, for instance, with a laugh, "Are the spears still hanging on the ceiling?" On his thirtieth birthday the grandmother and Werner invited his father and girlfriend, me, and two other carers from his childhood to celebrate. We were witness to an adult life that had found a kind of calm; witnesses also to the loneliness of the grandmother and grandson, now of thirty years standing.

A few weeks ago Werner called me to thank me after the letter on his thirty-seventh birthday. He told me how he had reacted to his grandmother's stroke. He had not at first understood what was happening but had then called for help. As a result of the stroke she could no longer get out of bed and it was difficult to understand what she was saying. Someone came by, morning and evening, from the mobile nursing service and his father's girlfriend looked after things, and Werner himself was still living in the house alone with her. During the day he was at work, which he quite liked; only at the weekends it was boring. How many months things had been like this he couldn't tell me. He only had a subjective feeling about the time: "It's been like this for ages." In this conversation he spoke for the first time about his awareness of growing old. "Joachim, you wouldn't recognise me. Just imagine, I'm sitting here wearing a nosebike" (jokey term for spectacles). We arranged that I would pick him up soon so he could see the new outpatients premises and the old colleagues he could remember.

We lack the intimacy today of the old relationship of shared play and talk which would have enabled him to confide and communicate what it meant to him to be someone who wore spectacles, an adult growing older and having to deal with fears, losses, and tensions. In the old days he had been a great robber of others' spectacles who had had to rid himself of his own inner terror by terrorising others and had to fill his mental-emotional gaps with *autistic objects* which were related in shifted form to lost love *objects*. What Werner learnt with us and we with him went beyond forms of suffering and reflection. We all gained.

### Miriam, adolescent to mother

When Miriam joined us she was sixteen years old and had broken off two attempts at finishing her schooling. Before coming she had been supported over years by an institution that cooperates with our Verein but which saw no further possibilities of helping her to get a school qualification. We were approached because this institution knew of our "into-work project" and hoped if Miriam was closely "accompanied" new perspectives for her might be developed with her.

## The into-work project

The into-work project is a concept for young people starting at a very basic level to help them get accustomed to conditions in school and working life. Originally conceived of as a structure for morning activity and development of perspectives for those living in our Hagenwört group home, since 2003 there has also been a weekly programme for people in outpatient treatment aiming to acquire the most basic abilities associated with work, namely, getting up in the morning, arriving punctually at work, concentrating on work for two hours, keeping to given times for breaks, using public transport etc.

With this as our basis we think about what direction further vocational development might take. If it is a question of further schooling we work closely with the school for young patients at the University Clinical Centre in Tübingen where some of our clients can take an examination within the framework of the Vocational Preparation Year at the level of the school leaving certificate from a *Hauptschule* (Level 2 Unesco (ISCED)). In addition we try to find out with the clients what kind of work can be considered by accompanying them in work experience placements. Questions come up such as "Can I stick it through an eight-hour day?", "Is waitressing still going to be my dream job after one week?", "How do I get on with colleagues?"

The process of bringing dreams into line with reality and above all of looking seriously at the client's own illness-based impairments is extremely painful. The most important thing for us is to let the young people gather their own experience. Saying "You'll never manage that" has seldom had a good effect. The consideration of their individual wishes is crucial. With this in mind we develop individually adapted settings that are appropriate to the client's needs and at the same time try to further a development leading out of our premises into the world outside.

## From work project to supported living in a young people's group home

Miriam was still living with her mother at the outset of our work with her and spent her time mainly at her boyfriend's place during the day, although daytime is not really the right word here. Miriam's days usually began around five in the afternoon, running into the small hours. To expect her to turn up for a meeting at three in the afternoon was asking too much of her. In a very short time the situation at home with

Miriam's mother escalated to the point that—when we were officially approached—it was already a question of a "whole package": Miriam was to be supported not only in finding a line of work or getting a school qualification but also in learning to live independently.

At our first encounter Miriam sat next to her carer in silence. She said practically nothing. When we spoke about our forms of support she said: "I can't do more than one appointment a week, it's too much for me, it's always been like this with me, you can ask my carer, more is no go."

In the following weeks it soon turned out that Miriam did not turn up for appointments in which it was a question of "just" cooking and getting to know one another. Mostly she overslept and did not answer phone calls. All the appointments, however, that were concerned with looking for a flat, filling in forms, or buying things for the new flat were a different matter. She appeared punctually at these. These activities at first took up a lot of time and energy and Miriam pressed for more appointments in order to deal with everything that needed doing. The Vocational Preparation Year we had suggested and discussed with her soon became unnecessary as she had been to the job centre on her own and signed on for a preparatory vocational course. Adjusting our *setting* to Miriam's needs and adapting the proposed relationship to her sensitivities proved, on looking back, to have been critical to making a good start in supporting her.

## Money

The first period was marked by fierce battles over Miriam's money. While we were under pressure to ensure there would still be something to eat in the fridge at the end of the month in order to guarantee the basic provisions for her first attempt at independent living, Miriam went to her mother with complaints that we were letting her freeze because we had refused her the money for a winter coat. My male colleague could not get over the feeling of being exploited at first. While he was being fiercely attacked and railed at over the payments of money, she kept our relationship free of these aggressive outbreaks. If we had not had regular supervision to accompany the process in which these *splittings* were worked through again and again he would probably have given up at this stage.

With the help of this arrangement and also with more information on her life history we were able to understand her anger with "the man" and so we tolerated the *splitting* and used it actively. So my colleague took over the thankless tasks of setting boundaries, negotiating money affairs, for example, while I was kept a bit free of these everyday concerns. As a result I was able to concentrate on the task of building a relationship with her which needed to be strong enough to sustain difficult situations. Apart from pragmatic viewpoints such as covering for holidays and absence through illness, this was the most important reason for not taking on this client alone but rather as a small team, as a pair of carers, since otherwise the danger of the project being broken off during the moments of her fierce, contemptuous attacks would have been great.

Allowing the *splitting* and with it the moments which I could experience as useful and beneficial also helped to prevent my colleague from seeing his work as hopeless and devoid of meaning. He was able to tolerate the violent emotions she showed him above all because they were interpreted in the framework of the supervision—in other words were connected with the anger Miriam felt towards her father—and were not taken by us as aggression directed against the person of my colleague.

Around the topic of money a pattern of behaviour emerged early on that has persisted in a problematic manner right through our support for Miriam till the present. Miriam possessed and still possesses no mental-emotional means of deferring needs which she experiences as existential. If the gratification of a need was not instantly met, for instance a cigarette she wanted to smoke, a particular food she wanted to eat, she would become terribly restless and aggressive. If at that moment the refusal to gratify her desire could be blamed on a person she would attack him violently, whether he was responsible or not.

If one connects this inability of the parent to postpone the gratification of his or her own urgent wishes with the necessity of subordinating them to the needs of a child, one can see what grave difficulties can result in providing for a child. If this inability in a parent to contain his or her own feelings collides with the child's emotions that require containment, then a highly charged atmosphere can develop in a family.

## Life—it would happen!

A tragic accident in Miriam's close circle of acquaintances changed her radically. After it happened she suffered from states of acute fear and could not be left alone for a moment. She was very open in her contacts with us and willing to talk but during this time she dropped out of the vocational course she had started. She withdrew into her boyfriend's family and broke off the vocational preparation course.

Although we continued to offer Miriam socio-therapeutic, one-to-one sessions she was not able to accept this framework of regular appointments. Instead what developed in our next setting were very serious conversations about her fears, her life history, and the connection between her fear and what she had experienced. Above all in the car, speaking casually, and not speaking directly about the main subjects, it became possible to talk about her inner themes. We often sat in front of the bank or some shop and couldn't get out straight away because we needed to carry on the conversation begun while driving.

These intense conversations very seldom took place more than once a week. It seemed to Miriam to be too close and to become too threatening. Work on uncovering themes was only possible to a limited degree since many of those that came up at this time were too painful for her. In this work we respected the boundaries she set as being what she could tolerate. The setting, which was built around her everyday needs, allowed her to keep control over the intensity and frequency of these conversations. Inner themes and hardships alternated with everyday concerns. It seemed that it was only in the shift back and forth between inner to outer that she could turn to interstates, to her most personal inner fears, needs, and thoughts.

In the midst of this Miriam became pregnant. The initial reaction to this situation was that she did not seem in good shape for a pregnancy either physically or in mental-emotional terms. But on the other hand the pregnancy relieved her of certain pressures. Through the repeated breaking off of her vocational preparation course, her school and vocational career had become more difficult and the pregnancy opened up a completely new perspective for her. Her great worry was whether we could remain her familiar people to turn to, since we would no longer be supporting her on her path into the world of work. A shift of responsibilities in the area of financial support for her—she now received assistance from the job centre and no longer from the local authority young people's services—expressed the transition from adolescent to adult in symbolic form. Here we were very lucky to find our view strongly supported by the staff member at the local authority young people's services. This made it possible—particularly now over this major change in Miriam's life—to keep up the relationships that had developed with us and were now very stable. In this way many things changed in formal terms—the project of supported accommodation was changed first into intensive socio-pedagogic help, and then after the birth of the child into family assistance. The benefit payments for her living costs now came from the job centre—but the concrete support in everyday matters was covered by the same carers.

### Brief review

As a small child Miriam had lived for a long time in various women's refuges. Her father was an alcoholic and her mother had been violently treated by him. Although she does not remember much about this time it is most likely the case that inwardly her mother was not really able to focus on her children but was preoccupied with getting out of her dire position. Fear must have played a large part in Miriam's early life. There was the constant threat of violence, the flight from home, being discovered in the women's refuge, then flight again. Then the arrival in a strange town and the slow building up of a new life, which at first must have been marked by a lack of basic necessities. With the lack of food, furniture, and supportive structures it must have taken a long time till a new rhythm of life was found. How was a young woman like Miriam, who had herself received so little love and attention, going to be able to give her own child the necessary attention and care? Despite this experience of deprivation one could sense a capability to form relationships there which came out in stable though complicated relationships both with her family and with her boyfriend of many years, the father of the child.

In the actual work of supporting her this biography and background meant that alongside the fears already described the worry kept recurring that her daughter Alessa, though sufficiently provided for materially might not receive enough attention and might have to subordinate her life to that of an erratic young person. How was a young mother who was herself at times overwhelmed by fears and was still fighting to *contain* her own undigested feelings going to be able to bear the emotions of a small child? And what form of support could one imagine for the mother that would enable her to look after her child sufficiently well—emotionally?

### In two minds: which is the child needing care?

Already during her pregnancy the focus of our responsibility shifted. From now on it was our concern to keep not only Miriam's development in view but also the healthy development of the growing child inside her. Before the pregnancy the fact that she was underweight had been a marginal topic–although in the battles over how she used her money it had in the end become about feeding herself properly. Now eating healthy and above all sufficient food was vital for the unborn child. Her lack of appetite and failure to buy fresh, vitamin-rich food formed a large part of our concern and the time spent with her. As regards money she had decided despite our expressed qualms to take over the management of her money herself after the source of it was shifted to the job centre. Suddenly it was no longer a question of satisfying Miriam's own needs but of balancing her needs with those of the child. Whereas before we had been emphatically on Miriam's side we now found ourselves caught up in the tension between mother and daughter. After Alessa's birth this expansion of concern was mirrored in a change at the formal level.

Initially the care plan had been formulated in Miriam's name with her development and health as the focus of our work. Now the measure was rewritten as one for Alessa. In direct relationship work this change had great significance. The "well-being" of the child had previously referred to Miriam but now she was the mother to be counselled for the well-being of her as yet unborn child. In this outward double focus Miriam's inner ambivalence towards her child was shown. On the one hand she wanted and wants to look after her child well and wants perhaps also to recompense her own inner, injured child. On the other hand, feelings of envy appeared as did the wish to be fed and looked after instead of having to do the looking after herself since she had not been sufficiently cared for emotionally as a child.

What was very positive was that Miriam concerned herself with many aspects of becoming a mother in a serious and realistic way. She knew she was subject to violent outbreaks of feeling and was anxious that she might not be able to calm her baby. And we were equally anxious, a fact that expressed itself in rather too large a present when Alessa was born, an electrically driven crib supposed to help restless babies go to sleep. She regularly read about the development of the baby in the womb in a booklet her gynaecologist had given her, assiduously following the growth of the new life inside her. She attended all appointments in the programme of medical check-ups, looking forward to each appointment and above all to the first "photos" of her daughter. As regards finances she had become "sensible" and even though money management has remained difficult the expected catastrophe has not occurred. She began to plan her expenditure. After a time marked by a certain amount of financial chaos, which was, however, more connected with external factors than with her behaviour, there has not been a single day in which she was not able to provide for herself and her daughter.

The focus on the child always involved a certain balancing act. We would often have a strong sense that we needed to keep Miriam's needs in view and not concern ourselves too much with Alessa since Miriam could only look after her child well if given good emotional support herself. Did turning to the child mean our turning away from her? Often the two sets of needs came into collision. Miriam frequently experienced the needs of the small child with her demand for instant satisfaction as an attack on herself. It was constantly necessary to accept the two sets of needs as being equally important, to create a space for Miriam herself, and nevertheless insist on her understanding that this small baby was not yet capable of waiting for her needs to be satisfied.

The main function of our intensive care during this period was to offer *containment* for Miriam's marked fears. Alongside this came the practical support of accompanying her to doctors' appointments, shopping, and looking for a larger flat. Our supervision sessions mirrored our own great fears. How were we going to prevent the baby from getting hurt in an outbreak of emotion? How would we be able to influence the situation in such a way that Alessa would be able to grow up in a good environment?

## Working along the lines of defence

It was only by working in accordance with Miriam's wishes as to the degree of involvement, by changing and adapting the setting to her individual needs, that we were able to form a relationship strong enough to work through difficult moments and conflicts without endangering the care plan itself. A client has to have great trust to let professional helpers come into her own family and to allow someone who was originally a stranger to see her very personal fears and difficulties. The situation is different from that of a psychotherapeutic relationship. With us there is close connection to the *Jugendamt*, the local authority children and young people's services, and our function is therefore a good deal more complicated and two-edged. Although we are primarily considered as helping agents it is also our task to make sure that the child's development is healthy. If the child is endangered—and such situations are not always as obvious as severe neglect (there could be lack of hygiene or insufficient food), or if there is any abuse the authorities have to be informed of the situation. In addition to regular meetings over care plans there is cooperation with the *Jugendamt* which is quite openly made clear to clients. Our work takes place in this area of dynamic tension between care and control.

Just once I had to rush to Miriam and take over Alessa when Miriam called in a state of exhaustion, having had no sleep and not knowing what to do because Alessa had been crying for hours. This "allowing us to see her" when she was at the end of her tether, allowing us to help but hand back maternal competence to her straight afterwards, was an important point in the course of the care we offered her.

## A few concluding remarks

With closeness and regular contact of this kind there is always a danger of being "swallowed up" in the family dynamics through powerful identification processes and of not retaining enough detachment and professional distance to be able to remain effective in the special role of professional helper. In this situation working as a pair of carers was an important regulatory factor as was having frequent and regular supervision. Having the outsider's view and persistent questioning of one's own work made it possible to work this close to the client and yet keep the necessary distance.

Often the children and young people's services are only able to intervene when things have already gone too far and the situation has escalated; intervention is thereby made difficult. It would make sense for there to be more focus in this field on the early relationships between parents and children before difficulties crop up to prevent the passing on from generation to generation of existing negative patterns of behaviour and to foster healthier ones. It remains to be seen if that will happen for Alessa.

Recently Miriam has returned to school. This has happened without any pressure from outside. She had developed a desire to get school qualifications. So alongside baby-care, the school and the into-work project are back in demand and she can be supported by the carers she knows.

## Gustav

### Acting, thinking, understanding

The young people new to the Hagenwört group learn that they are going to have to be involved in more than just being in the group home. To stay there they also have to go out. We expect them to be prepared to fit into a school or place of work as well as living in this beautiful old house. The staff of our into-work project are there to help them and if needed are available for intensive support during this integration and in the transitions that are part of it. And they are also required to engage in a therapeutic process with another person they will meet at our out-patient rooms in Tübingen and who has nothing to do with the every-day processes in the group home.

Regular individual case supervision sessions are held with the members of staff of these separate places which make very different demands on the clients and which frequently stimulate very different levels of the clients' mental-emotional development. From the start we concentrate on using three locations: the place of everyday life, the place of school and work, and the place of therapy, and this helps us to make space available for the individual, delusional world of a resident and still not let reality out of sight.

A young man I'm going to call Gustav was admitted here after he had been treated over a year in a child and adolescent psychiatric unit. He had kept the ward busy there with marked compulsive behaviour concerning going to the toilet and frequent bed-wetting. There was no way of setting up a reasonable working alliance with his mother who suffered from a mental-emotional disorder. His father lived at a great distance and his relations with Gustav had been broken off. No one quite knew what to do with the sixteen-year-old. There was no prospect of schooling and it was at this stage that we received an application for admission here.

Gustav wanted to come to us to "move on" and to free himself of his compulsive behaviour and live a normal life. In the first phase we—a little euphorically—were going to lead him, with strict structuring, into a life outside the walls of the psychiatric hospital and far from the world of delusions he was trapped in with his mother. Gustav was happy to agree to this. Looking back one can ask whether he hadn't perhaps pro-jected onto us his feelings of hope and was to be regarded as the initia-tor of our spirit of optimism.

We deliberately and consistently took no notice of his compulsions concerning toilet matters and only confronted him with the consequences if he was upsetting his routine for the day or disturbing the other residents.

Working with the mother proved difficult and finally the relationship was broken off. This had something to do with the fact that we had made contact with Gustav's father and were building this up carefully. Gustav and his father began to see each other regularly. Gustav said he was glad not to see his mother any more and to get to know his father now. We had the impression he was taking in all our ideas and suggestions gratefully. He went to his therapy sessions regularly, went fairly reliably to a school in which a special structure had been worked out for him, and he kept saying how important it was for him to work with us carers in the group home. Only somehow working together became less and less successful and arguments with him became more frequent and fiercer. He was caught smoking on our balcony although we have a ban on smoking in the house and for him smoking was expressly completely forbidden. He hung around the female residents and reacted aggressively if we interfered in these close contacts out of our obligation to look after the welfare of all residents. He often answered brusquely to concerns of ours and was quick to take offence.

In our *countertransference* phantasies what often cropped up was the wish to make it clear to him, forcefully, why he was here, or then again there would be a resigned realisation that we could not give him the structure he needed. In attempts to talk to him we were left with the feeling that we had been talking at cross purposes. Often it was not even possible to greet him without his making some kind of insulting remark. Sometimes Gustav would not return a friendly hello, or at other times he would return the greeting nicely, pat us on the shoulder, or even hug us. In most encounters we felt provoked and often reacted correspondingly curtly, whereupon he would feel misunderstood by us.

In one supervision, after we had given vent to our sense of discontent and among other things had come up with the idea that Gustav should be sent to the clinic for a few days—even if only for disciplinary reasons, we managed to focus more clearly on what he was trying to do, on what we expected, and on this mismatch of conceptions. Gustav had left the child and adolescent psychiatric hospital because he wanted to be normal here with us.

The contact with his mother had broken off and he did not want ever to be like her. He wasn't mad, as he told us! He wanted to be a normal boy of his age and even if this did not quite work straightaway at least he wanted to become normal quickly. And we realised the longer we lived with him how ill he was and how little he had developed abilities to make social contacts and relationships.

Supervision became a struggle to find possible ways to get into contact with the sick and delusional sides of Gustav and to let something of this appear in our contacts with him. This meant trying to set up a genuine relationship with him—beyond setting boundaries, beyond any educational task or responses to his provocations—a relationship which might enable him to reach the deeply wounded sides of his inner life.

On the day after the supervision he was not in the dining room at supper time. I went to look for him in his room and asked him to come to table. He answered in a friendly way and said he was just coming, but then he didn't come. It wasn't until the end of supper that he turned up and accepted my invitation to come to my office afterwards with a puzzled look. The fact that I did not reproach him but was interested to hear what made it so difficult for him to join us for supper just increased his bewilderment. When I put myself in his shoes and said I was think-ing it must perhaps depress him if he wanted to be there for supper and couldn't manage it, he was nonplussed and thoughtful. Clearly he wasn't used to the experience of being spoken to with empathy.

It is going to take many such encounters to relax Gustav's *defences* and help him to work via these encounters towards an understanding and acceptance of what his needs are. He is boycotting himself, refus-ing to have dealings with himself, and delegating this boycott to others with the result that they won't have dealings with him.

Gaining such insight would be an important step in detaching from the pathological relationship with his mother. He will continue to try to provoke us so that we attack him—this then being a confirmation of his expectation of being attacked, punished, and constrained. Our reflection on the relation to him and the resulting new experiences for him—because we shall not fulfil his expectations—will however gradu-ally enable him to change.

## Jonas and the hole in his soul

"I think I have a hole in my soul …" Jonas spoke these words in tears. Before that, in a stormy scene with a member of staff he had been screaming as if ready to die. Jonas was admitted to the therapeutic home in Rottenburg at age thirteen and a half. The following account describes scenes from the first years of our encounter with him (see also Grohmann, Gschwender, & Schmidt, 1993; Schmidt, 1995).

## On his previous history

Jonas grew up as the only child of his single mother. His biological father and his mother separated when he was two and a half. Between the ages of four and five he lived with his mother in Greece for a year, in a hut on the beach. Stories of this time give the impression of an Eden-like togetherness. The time that followed in Germany was experienced as a rift. Repeatedly, because of accidents and operations on Jonas he experienced encounters with hospitals and doctors as times of being overpowered. Jonas said they had wanted to take him away from his mother at birth. Situations of separation and other real and imaginary and symbolic operations all carried elements of violent breaks. Isolated, clinging to each other, mother and child survived seemingly threatening incisions in their lives. The appearance of any third person in the Robinson Crusoe scenario—except for the ambivalent figure of the doctor, hardly seems to have happened. Any partners for the mother withdrew after a short time. The mother often felt she had to choose between the partner or Jonas. The men in question had not felt able to take on Jonas.

When he was ten the school also felt it could not cope with Jonas. They were advised to put him in a home but the mother could not bring herself to agree to this. Jonas began to wander from home, truanting, visiting slaughterhouses where he picked up sheep's heads and cows' eyes which he took home or took to school to frighten others with. Finally Jonas took himself to the doctor and told him about his suicidal phantasies.

He was admitted to a remedial institution. After five weeks he was expelled: he had broken out and had tried to find his way back to his mother. Among other things he had threatened the small children of the members of staff and threatened his mother that he would commit suicide. After this he landed in a child and adolescent psychiatric hospital.

The children's ward turned out not to be secure enough and he was moved to the adolescent ward. After over a year they saw no further possibilities for development for him in their framework.

*First encounters—enjoying shock*

My first encounter with Jonas on his first visit to the home was with his mother. Jonas was of medium height, and like his mother he had long blond hair and wore glasses. The clothes he wore were loose-cut and his body appeared thin and fragile in them. He didn't make direct eye contact, his face was pale and unexpressive. With his mouth and hands, which he held knotted together, he kept making stereotype movements. He was afraid of any physical contact. In the therapy room he discovered a child's doctor's bag that attracted his attention instantly. He opened it, went straight for the syringe, grabbed his mother's arm, looked expertly for a vein, and gave her an injection in front of my very eyes—quite roughly. Unlike me the mother did not seem to be a bit taken aback by this doctor game and she let him do what he wanted.

I was disconcerted by this kind of treatment. On the day he was admitted Jonas appeared with infusion tubes in his nose secured with plasters which he had applied himself "for protection". In his hand he carried a home-made doctor's bag in cardboard which he had been given as a farewell present by the child and adolescent psychiatric hospital.

Right from the beginning Jonas peppered us with questions. When could he go home? When would his mother visit him? What would happen if he ran away? If he hurt himself or other people or exposed himself to risky situations? Did they hit you in this home? What happened if a child injured another child or a member of staff? Did we have scalpels, syringes, and tubes here? His phantasies of running away were connected with a lively interest in where the slaughterhouses were in the neighbourhood, pictures of blood, dead animal heads, and body parts. He described in terrifyingly graphic detail how animals were killed with a cattle gun and how their bodies were hung up headless on hooks, with pools of blood under them. I was deeply shocked and disconcerted by these stories. In the first days with us Jonas would only go around with the infusion tubes in his nose and the doctor's bag in his hand. He wanted them with him even outside the house. After a few days he was able to leave them in his room.

After that he no longer stuck to the tubes, but he stuck to *us*. In an unbroken stream of speech he flooded us with his phantasies and questions. He ordered us not to speak. Our speaking, our voices and looks seemed to threaten him physically. Words such as *you*, *no*, and *blood* were not allowed in his presence. They triggered in him "disturbance feelings", which made themselves felt at particular points in the body: "Nose is disturbing me", "Eye is twitching".

He would hold his hands over his ears saying "Don't want to hear that", or threatened to kick the other person in the face. He also had compulsive "habits"—making smacking noises with his tongue, biting himself as he did so inside his cheek, lip smacking and grimaces, glottal clicking, clicking in the mouth and lip area, and hearing sounds in his ears. Without being able to connect a particular feeling with these sounds from points in the body he would stand in front of us and ask, "Does that sound high or low?"

As if he was without any protective skin everything was "too close", "too much" for him and sent him into a panic. He flailed around or hit himself on the head. The break times when he was expected to be in his room were almost too much for him. At night he had to have the sound of a radio. If he was left to himself "pictures" would come up of the slaughterhouse, of dead cows and blood.

Two days before his mother's second visit to the home Jonas managed to inject a medicine into the hands and arms of two other residents. This shocked us in itself, but additionally because despite our knowing about his acting-out and despite our raised awareness and attention to him, he had managed to put his phantasies into action. Jonas was on the one hand relieved his act had been discovered but was nervous about possible consequences. We took his syringes away from him, and everything else that might be dangerous found in his room. It was only later that we discovered he had never been given these utensils by the clinic but had filched them from the ward.

Apart from increasing his medication we set up an almost constant surveillance. We hoped alongside concrete external protective measures that Jonas would begin to bind his phantasies and fears in the one-to-one sessions with me and would thus be able to deal with them in an arena away from everyday life.

Jonas returned from his first weekend at home with an infusion tube stuck into his arm. He and his mother had given each other infusions, he explained. Shortly after that his mother planned to go on a three-week holiday. She informed us that Jonas was in possession of tablets. She hadn't taken them away from him. We then found them in Jonas room alongside syringes and other dangerous objects he had brought with him from home. We took them into safe keeping. The next morning

Jonas ran away from the home and was picked up later by the police at the slaughterhouse. There he had wanted to see "dead cows and blood" and fetch "cows' eyes" he told us. Later that afternoon he managed in an unnoticed moment to cut defenceless female patients in the arm and neck with pieces of broken glass. His comment was that he never wanted to see his mother again.

Jonas had managed to force us to set up similar arrangements to those in the psychiatric clinic. We had put bars on the windows and doors. In the same way as we controlled and followed his every step, he controlled and followed ours—outwardly and inwardly. As time went by, however, he was able to stabilise himself. He now turned to us when "pictures came". In these moments he wanted us to hold him for a short while. A few months later the phantasies of running away returned. In fact he did run away again one night or maybe early morning, escaping by a window. He found his way to his mother, taking with him a bloody sheep's head he had somehow wangled from the slaughterhouse. He was going to boil it up and fry the eyes.

Once Jonas lifted a window from its hinges on the first floor and let it drop down onto the street. In doing so he was not only attacking the body frame of the house but was also depriving himself of protection. Jonas: "My mother doesn't want me any more." At this time a new life partner moved in with his mother. Jonas seemed to be expressing the existential loss of his place with his mother in this action.

## A different arena

Half a year later the situation had calmed down a little. Jonas was now able to *say* something about his actions *after the event*. He had wanted to be thrown out of the home and go back to his mother, into the psychiatric hospital, or into prison. But now he didn't want to get out. He said he was glad to be in the home, he seemed to feel "held" there. In the one-to-one sessions he lay down in a hammock and I was to rock him. He even asked me to sing to him while he swung there. He no longer just covered his ears with his hands when I spoke but would occasionally say "Nonsense" or "Rubbish". Feeling secure and "rocked in safety" he began to enjoy playing that he was falling out of the hammock—asking also whether I would hold him or let him fall.

Growing bolder now, Jonas wanted to extend this game. He let himself be wheeled around by me in the wheelbarrow out in the garden of the home. He discovered a pleasure in playing with the idea of falling out. Then he wanted to leave the safe haven of the garden and carry the game out into the street. With some hesitation I let this happen. So we often went down like this to the river Neckar. It was as if I was wheeling a small child around in a pram. He wanted to be rocked in the wheelbarrow, cocooning himself at times trustingly in a blanket, pulling it over his head, and trusting me to hold on to him and get him back home safely. At times he became daring and wanted to take over the steering. He wanted to wheel me: he would have enjoyed wheeling me into the Neckar. Here I drew the line (my line!) and told him he wasn't there to hold me. After all, I had the responsibility for him and also that nothing happened to him or me and that nothing should go off the rails. I was thinking of the accidents that Jonas had had. Jonas asked, "Will you hold me or will you let me fall?", "Who has to hold whom?", "Who is the adult, who is the child?"—but he also began to ask about a "third person" and about the law, indicating he was entering a psychic state of *triangulation*.

Before the summer holidays Jonas and his mother suddenly had the idea of spending a three-week holiday on an island in the Mediterranean. Jonas above all connected this idea with a memory of "then", an imagined untroubled Eden-like time, naked on the beach.

The familiar one-to-one session down by the Neckar changed. Jonas got out of the wheelbarrow and played that he had reached a border—a crossing-point at the border. I had to be the official at the border and check his papers. To my request for his passport and question where he wanted to go he said he had no passport but that he absolutely had to go to his mother; she was on holiday on the other side of the border. I said to him that I couldn't let him cross the border because he didn't have a valid passport. I was *not* to let him cross. That was part of the game. I had to make sure he didn't cross over and if necessary hold him back physically if he tried to get over without permission. He wanted to play this again and again. Independently of this his mother told us in a parental interview about a dream she had had. In this dream she was travelling in a train and came to a border where the official asked her for her papers. But her passport was out of date and the official wouldn't let her go through although she told him she absolutely had to get there to her son on the other side of the border.

Jonas played out what his mother had dreamt in the reality of his game. It was a little uncanny. In Jonas's game and in the mother's dream the psychic situation of mother and son was very clearly depicted: the imperative wish to go to the other and the *denial* or attempt to get around the border and the separation between them.

As well as being attracted by the idea of boundless regression Jonas was also scared of it. Over a weekend at home there were arguments with his mother. Jonas wanted to return to the home in Rottenburg and when his mother did not let him do so straightaway Jonas kicked her in the face. Shortly after that he secretly cut off his pubic hair that was just beginning to grow. He developed a swelling in the genital area. A hernia was diagnosed. All these things created the impression that a holiday for Jonas with his mother without a protective third person was too threatening. For Jonas himself the hospital appeared to be a phantasy rescuing him from his dilemma. The hernia did not have to be operated on instantly but there was the danger that if they went on holiday he might have to have an emergency operation. In this way the decision was reached and agreed by all that Jonas was to have the operation instead of the holiday. The nearer the date of the operation came the greater his fear of the operation grew. In our sessions he wanted to play the scene in which he was brutally and if necessary against his will overwhelmed by the doctors—whom I was to represent; they were to pin him down and operate on him despite all his screams, with him squirming in resistance.

Finally, with us accompanying him throughout the operation which was done in day surgery, it all went very well. Jonas's room in the home was set up as the sick room. He was able to let himself be nursed, fed, and washed with relatively little fear. He was able to enjoy it without feeling attacked at his physical boundary. Only when the stitches were taken out did he show fear. He thought the scar might "break open" or "tear open".

Finally he gave the scar a loving name: he called it "baby-scar". Shortly before Christmas when it was a question again of whether he should go home he produced a similar scenario around a second hernia. Christmas at home had to make way for a second operation. What remained after that was a "mother-scar". It seemed the scars were closing something, holding something together. Jonas seemed at this point to feel more represented by these "wound-marks" written onto his body than by his given name. During the day, it was like a tic, he would pull up his shirt to look at these scars to make sure they were holding as if in fear that something might "break through" if under too much pressure.

He developed problems with the various "sensitive" points of his body one after the other. As a result we visited all kinds of doctors. Jonas's body was "explored", examined, and treated a number of times. He had bitten regular holes in his mouth by chewing the inside of his cheek. Inflammations or damage to the eyes, ears, penis, and anus required treatment as well. His idea was that something had to be removed from his body in an operation for him to feel better. In this spirit he wanted to go to the ear, nose, and throat clinic to have his adenoids removed. He hoped that his feelings of disturbance might disappear with this operation.

Increasingly the question now came up of what might emerge in place of these feelings and habits. What would it be like if they weren't there? On the one hand Jonas wanted to be rid of them because they caused him suffering but on the other hand he was attached to them and was afraid they might be taken away from him. They seemed to fill an inner space where there might otherwise be an unbearable void and non-aliveness.

## The shock of enjoyment

A recurring question was whether Jonas was to go home at the weekend or not. He hadn't been home for a considerable time now. At this time he had a phantasy of killing his mother: by Jewish kosher slaughter, cutting off her head. Jonas "had to" go home, claiming his mother "didn't mind". But who was to decide? Was it good for him to go home? Was it dangerous? Could we take the responsibility if he went?

I brought up these questions in supervision. I did not always want to have to decide and be in the position of having the last word. I was really tired of this role of always having to know what was right. It was becoming intolerable, it was too much for me, I wanted to pass the buck. For an hour the talk went back and forth in the session without any result. One supervisor finally remarked just before the close it was "all a bit cerebral". As no real decision had been made I said rather angrily "I'm sick of this silly game between Jonas and his mother—this eternal back and forth." This clear heartfelt statement became our criterion for a decision. What further course things would take only became clear to me in a second supervision that evening, in a *case production* (on the method of case production cf. Amuser-Burger, 1994). There I repeated the questions I had put in the afternoon. But here I was allowed to delegate these questions to someone else who—put in my place—had to justify himself. The discussion that followed without my having to take part in it showed people were moved. It was first of all a relief for me to be able simply to listen without having to take any real action. And in me, too, things moved back and forth following the path of the discussion.

Positions were taken up and then changed again, against the mother or against Jonas, and many felt the need to be stricter. When at the end I had to say how I had felt while listening I said I felt I was being treated unfairly when they had all been attacking one side or another. Faced with their closed ranks I had felt very lonely. I remembered how Jonas had always used the words "I don't want it to be my fault. I'm being treated unfairly." It was only now that I could feel with real affect what loneliness, isolation, and exclusion was hidden behind these words. His experience had become *my* loneliness—within the team too. The perverse pleasure which Jonas had drawn from my laying down the law seemed to serve the same end: it meant that he did not have to feel this loneliness, and could ward off this pain and grief. And later he could proclaim some different "*No!*" that would not entail the fear of being completely wiped out, the fear of a radical break.

## *So far …*

What path had we travelled? I could see three stages. At first the nameless dread—the endless state of shock—was in the foreground, and it was a question of realising a form of holding and *containing* through our actions—with reference to Jonas's physical self and to the structure of the framework. In his stagings in the real world Jonas acted out what he could not symbolise between the extreme states of absolute dissolution and absolute insulation, between the wish for complete closure and control and regression without borders of any kind. We responded to his stagings by creating a closed framework with concrete measures and in a way formed a protection against stimuli with our physical presence.

In a second phase the one-to-one sessions took on greater importance. The phantasies and fears increasingly became the object of our encounter and the relationship between Jonas and myself. In this I saw myself exposed in an almost unbearable way to what were at times Jonas's boundless demands and was challenged by them. Also the space which developed between the mother and Jonas—the untaken space—was now there for me to be the representation of a border, a stopgap. It was only in the last phase that we were no longer stopping up holes and that something could remain open between Jonas and me. This increased as he became able to feel his pain, his grief, his "hole in the soul" and articulate it—to give birth to himself.

Jonas himself described the journey taken afterwards in his own way: "Can you believe it? I had a dream. I wanted to climb up a tower. But I had to go right deep down to the very bottom to get up to the top. Can you believe such a thing?"

# GLOSSARY

## Acting out

The term *acting out* refers to two different phenomena. Within psychoanalytic treatment the word refers to the reviving of repressed content in the sense of a *compulsion to repeat* as a disposition to act rather than to remember. Impulses and affects appear as actions in the *transference*, they are experienced by the patient and so made accessible to interpretation. *Acting out* in a second interpretation is a term describing how the patient departs from the rule of confining himself to talking in psychoanalytic treatment and resorts to physical action within or outside the therapy. Over time this meaning with its negative overtones has gained ascendance and the term has come to be understood to mean impulsive action of antisocial character, or action endangering the self or others.

With the growing understanding of *transference* and *countertransference* and insight into their mutual influence and dynamic character, *acting out* also on the part of the analyst, which is known as *enactment*, has shifted more into the centre of attention. This, too, is regarded on the one hand as being an inevitable part of the psychoanalytic process and as a source of live exchange between analyst and analysand but it is, on the other hand, also a factor which if it is not examined can sorely disturb the analysis, or indeed destroy it.

Psychoanalytic social work devotes a great deal of attention to *acting out*. The work is carried out in a setting of which precisely this inter-play of actions between social worker and client is the hallmark. It is often only possible after the event to reach conscious reflection on the *unconscious* meaning of such actions. The work of finding insight into *unconscious* determinants of the client's actions is predominantly devel-oped in the here and now of everyday life and in the conversations that accompany it. Because of their personality problems the clients are often significantly impaired in their ability to control impulses and *acting out*, as defined above. This is why well-reflected handling of action-based dealings with the clients, those in the form of *enactments* or of active adaption of the setting conditions to the client's abilities, is of central importance in psychoanalytic social work.

## Autistic defence/autistic object

Psychoanalysis seeks to understand autistic disorders and autistic symptom formations not mainly in terms of a disability, for instance in communication, interaction, and perception, but above all in the way such processes can be seen as psychologically functional in defending the person against anxieties. This is why one speaks of forms of *autistic defence* which all serve to avoid ways of experiencing that trigger vio-lent, psychotic fears. To do so a person insulates himself, so to speak creating a second skin and avoiding mental and emotional processes of exchange. In this context *autistic objects* take on importance. These are most often hard objects which have to be constantly available and which are used to insulate against the perception of things in the outer world and also for self-stimulation.

*Autistic objects* are experienced by the child as a part of the child's own body. In this way the child wards off experiences of separation and helplessness. *Autistic objects* have a self-soothing effect. Among other things, through sensory stimulation they offer a seemingly omnipotent control over external reality and thus a kind of mechanical reliability which can never be a quality of living *objects* (persons) because of their inherent spontaneity. From this understanding of the *autistic object* it will be clear that any socially appropriate use of the object would only disturb its real function for the client's inner balance (Gunter, 2006b; Tustin, 1990).

Social workers have to deal with this form of *defence* against a fear of relationships when they work with autistic clients and bear it in mind if they wish to develop an understanding of the often bizarre fixations of their clients on objects and on their wish to keep all parameters in their environment exactly as they are. This also involves an understanding of the resistance shown to any sort of change and the outbursts of aggression that accompany it. It is a question of balance: on the one hand there is the agenda of social pedagogy to support the client while also demanding something of him and, on the other hand, the importance of showing acceptance of his needs to protect and defend himself. Keeping the right balance between these two things is an art which is decisive for the success of the measure in question. Such manoeuvres directed against a live exchange in relationships are also found in a somewhat milder form in clients with personality disorders and in those in a state of social disintegration.

## Conflict and trauma

Psychoanalysis has always from the very beginning been a psychology of conflict. The conflicts with which it is concerned are psychic conflicts. Over the course of the development of psychoanalysis the views on where the conflicts lie have changed. Freud established the first model of conflict based on his treatment of women patients with hysteria in whom he regularly saw a sexual trauma in the background. The affect connected with it and all memories of it had been repressed because they were most embarrassing and distressing and conflicted with the person's sense of morality. Through fresh sexual experiences in adult life the earlier experiences were revived, the repressed content merged with them (see *deferred action*) and again evoked unbearable affects. The greater strength of sexual desire in the now adult person made complete repression—as was possible in childhood—now impossible, with the result that a compromise formation of repression and partial, *unconscious* satisfaction appeared in symptoms. Thus this first conflict model of Freud's was closely connected with a theory of trauma. What Freud regarded as a psychical trauma was an event that produced such a powerful increase in excitation in the inner life of a person in such a short time that the usual way of dealing with it failed, resulting in a continuing impairment of the ability to deal with stimuli and tension (1916–17, p. 284). In his early conception of hysteria, trauma lay in the seduction of the child by an adult and the accompanying flood of stimuli breaking in on the child. After Freud discovered the ubiquitous presence in children of sexual desire for their parents and had given up the theory of seduction the antagonists in the conflict changed. Now he placed ego drives and sexual drives in opposition to one another and the conditions of the conflict changed yet again with the introduction of the structural model (Freud, 1923b). This model now made it possible to describe conflict combinations between id and ego (drive versus reality principle), id and superego (drive versus morality/ideal), and ego and superego (demands of reality versus demands of the ideal). Likewise within an *agency*: this would be, for example, the ambivalence conflict of love and hate as the opposition of two drive tendencies, or within the superego the conflict between opposing norms, or again within the ego between contradictory *representations* of self or object. It is Freud's structural model of the mind combined with later elaborated theories of *object relations* that leads to new connections between trauma and conflict, since the intensified focus of the last decades on so-called early disorders and on post-traumatic stress disorder, stimulated essentially through work with survivors of the holocaust, has supplemented the psycho-economic trauma model of sensory overload with an object-relation model of trauma. In this model in severe traumatisations there is a breakdown both of the inner *object* relation between self and *object* and also of the communication between self- and *object* representations so important for a sense of security.

The *good, inner object* as mediator between self and environment falls silent, and the self has lost an empathic protective shield which had been provided by the internalised *primary object* (parent*).* After this loss the need for empathy is projected onto the perpetrator as the only available *object*. He or she is internalised as a malignant introject (Bohleber, 2008). An *identification with the aggressor* emerges.

From these trauma-associated psychic processes disparate concepts of the self, or *self-representations,* but also contradictory *object-representations* develop particularly if the trauma has been perpetrated by an *object* which should have promised protection, such as a parent.

A part of the inner psychic world is split off and withdrawn from consciousness because of its irreconcilability with the person's need to have a constant and coherent self. Usually it is the traumatised part, that part of the self which has developed from the unbearable experience of trauma, that is split off but it can also be the "good" part if the trauma was very extensive. In the latter case the client seems to be filled and almost totally identified with the destructive experience he suffered.

These psychic groupings are often found in clients of psychoanalytic social work. The majority of them have in their childhood and youth experienced traumatic relationships marked by maltreatment and abuse. In working with them, in an expression of an *unconscious compulsion to repeat* on the part of the client, the psychoanalytic social worker will find himself placed in the position of the abusing *object*. Feelings similar to those felt in the traumatic experience are now shown to the social worker and he will be unconsciously provoked also to become an abuser in reality; or the relations are turned around and the client takes the role of the *object* who abused him in the past and tries to force the psychoanalytic social worker into the role of victim. Both permutations are complicated because it is a question of trauma-induced and thus split-off internalised *object* and relationship *representations* which only become amenable to understanding and integration after a long period of work on the relationship. A thorough supervision is indispensable.

## Container-contained, containing

From Klein's description of *projective identification*, Bion developed a general concept of the relationship between *container* and *contained* in the human psyche. The very young child projects undigested and as yet undigestable psychic content, that is "raw bits of experience" (Bion) such as fear, anger, etc. (which Bion designated beta elements—using a mathematical term) into the mother ( = container). She digests these in her quiet attention to the child so that they acquire meaning (to which Bion gave the name alpha function). After this transformation the child can take the contents back into himself and work on them psychically, for instance in the form of thoughts.

The body itself and its functions can be seen as forms of the *container-contained* relationship (intake of food—digestion—excretion; breathing in and breathing out). It is however also a *container* for emotions and with the skin as the border between inside and outside it is a container in the literal sense of the word. The sexual act (penis—into—vagina) and even the fertilisation of the ovum by the sperm also follow this figure of thought. So it hardly comes as a surprise that such thoughts are often found in religious and philosophical systems. It is Bion's achievement not only to have related this way of seeing things to psychoanalytic terminology but also to have benefited clinical practice with his perceptions.

In social work it is important to realise that the processes in psychotic and other "primitive" psychic states can be better understood with the help of this model than via an analysis of their content. Moreover social and political systems, and indeed psychoanalytic social work itself with its sometimes complex setting constructions can also function as a *container*.

## Countertransference

(cf. Chapter Ten, *Transference—Countertransference—"Scene"*)

It was after his discovery of *transference* in psychoanalytic treatments that Freud detected *countertransference*. What he understood by this was the psychoanalyst's "unconscious sensing" of his patient. Freud saw the necessary neutrality of the analyst as being endangered by *countertransference* and demanded that the analyst should notice it and hold it down. The idea that *countertransference* was a disturbance of therapy was later replaced by the view that it is a specific response to the patient's *transference* and mirrors this. Heimann (1950) saw *countertransference* as induced by the patient. In current psychoanalysis two forms are represented: an extended perception and a narrower definition. The extended view of it regards all emotional reactions of the analyst to the patient as *countertransference*, the narrower definition sees only the affective reactions of the analyst to the *transference* induced by the patient as being *countertransference*. In particular it is the narrower definition which allows inferences to be drawn about the nature of the patient's *transference* and thus about *unconscious* parts of his inner world. The concept of *transference* and *countertransference* has been further developed into the intrapsychic taking over of roles and the acted dialogue. According to these concepts not only do intersubjective psychic processes take place between analyst and analysand but also interactional processes in which limited action occurs on both sides between the two, namely inter-*acting*. In such a relationship based on actions, internalised relationship patterns are played out as if on a stage. This happens particularly in the case of relationships belonging to an early biographical period of the patient's life before the development of *word presentations* (or mental images of words) and which are therefore represented in his inner world only in scenic form.

Like *transference, countertransference* and scenic acted dialogues are ubiquitous. They can therefore be found and used outside the psychoanalytic setting.

In psychoanalytic social work the awareness of *countertransference* and understanding of acted dialogues are particularly valuable because the clients in this setting usually have little ability to put inner processes and states into words. Often the only possible way to gain access to their inner world is the indirect path taken by the psychoanalytic social worker via the attunement to his own reactions. This is all the more useful because the clients often tend to present an image to the world of intimidating or pronounced independent behaviour intended to hide feelings of weakness and dependence.

## Compulsion to repeat

In clinical description *compulsion to repeat* denotes forms of behaviour, relationship combinations, formation of symptoms, and similar which repeat previous experience without this being conscious. In particular, repetition in psychoanalysis in the form of *transference* is of great significance in terms of treatment technique. Freud introduced the concept in "Remembering, Repeating and Working-Through" (1914g): "… we may say that the patient does not remember anything of what he has forgotten and repressed, but acts it out. He reproduces it not as a memory but as an action; he repeats it, without, of course, knowing that he is repeating it" (p. 149).

Later in "Beyond the Pleasure Principle" Freud (1920g) perceived the *compulsion to repeat* as more fundamental, as something which was inherent in every drive as an urge to regain an earlier state, and he connects it with the death drive he postulated. Debates on the various aspects of the *compulsion to repeat* continue to the present day.

In particular there is controversy over the question of whether the *compulsion to repeat*—as for instance in reactions to traumatisations (flashbacks, intrusions, repetitious dreams)—is to be seen rather as the attempt of the ego to deal with excessive tension (and so is to be regarded as a restitutive power) or whether it is the expression of a fundamental tendency towards disintegration.

For psychoanalytic social work it is significant that the *compulsion to repeat* is above all characterised by the fact that psychic contents are not thought but appear in actions. In modern neuroscientific reflections the reason for this is found in the fact that already in early childhood schemata of actions for the solution of emotional and interactional problems are stored in the *unconscious*, procedural memory and are reproduced in corresponding situations without any reworking through translation into language. They form the affective structure of the human psyche at the fundamental level and lead in a variety of ways, particularly in situations of stress, to a handing down of conflicts and corresponding modes of action from generation to generation.

## Defence

The concept of *defence* is a central element in psychoanalysis. Freud understood *defence* as the intrapsychic *defence* against the demands of the drives. In drive psychology *defence* was the opponent of the drive thus constituting a *psychic* conflict which might give rise to neurotic symptoms. The *defence* mechanism of *repression* was a particular focus of Freud's examination in his early studies on hysteria and anxiety neurosis. In his later theory of the structure of the psyche (Freud, 1923b) he located *defence*, seen as largely *unconscious*, in the ego. In Anna Freud's (1936) theory of *defence* and *defence* mechanisms, *defence* served not so much to control the drives as to master them appropriately. Her view of them extended their scope so that alongside mastering the drives the *defence* mechanisms came to be seen as a part of a person's character serving to deal with external reality.

The insights of *object relations* psychology and other more recent psychoanalytic theories have further extended the tasks of *defence*, alongside the control of drives, to include the regulation of affects and of interpersonal relationships. For instance, the experience of a state of unbearable grief can be delayed through postponement until it can be better tolerated and worked through, or a depression can be warded off with a so-called manic *defence* or with compulsive mechanisms.

The most important mechanism of interpersonal *defence* is *projective identification*, with the help of which an unacceptable aspect of the self is transposed to another person. Interpersonal *defence* can condense into an institutionalised *defence* (Mentzos, 1988) if there are institutionalised mechanisms, secured in rules, of drive-, affect-, and relationship control. In work with clients and patients suffering from early disorders (of which there are many among the clients of psychoanalytic social work), what regularly happens is that *defence* reactions against the relationship are aroused either in the patient or in the doctor or carer. If they have internalised destructive *object relationships*, patients may ward off relationships out of fear of a repetition of experiences of malignant relationships as manifests in autistic and schizoid phenomena. Also, from an unconscious fear of hard-to-bear entanglements in a therapeutic relationship, those treating them or caring for them may avoid such relationships, for instance, through external administrative measures.

## Deferred action

The concept of *deferred action* in Freud's work is part of his theory on the aetiology of neuroses. It describes the effect of an event being felt not at once but at a later time. Freud developed the concept in the explanation of the aetiology of hysteria (Kerz-Rühling, 1993). According to this, a sexually seductive event which is experienced at an early phase of development before sexual maturity has no pathogenic effect because it is not yet experienced and recognised as sexually significant. If at a later time, possibly not until after sexual maturity develops, that is after puberty, a similar event takes place, which in itself may be quite banal, then this experience merges with the earlier one and leads now to sexual confusion which can result in hysterical symptoms.

Hysterical neurosis is caused, in this view, by a series of events of which no single one on its own would create a neurosis. In this sense, *Nachträglichkeit*, *deferred action*, is the delayed effect of an early infantile event which makes itself felt through the *unconscious* merging of one or several later events.

A slightly different understanding, which assumes a circularity in psychic processes, emphasises the deferred investment of meaning in the event. This view is more widespread today. It is found in French psychoanalysis (Kerz-Rühling, 2008) in the work of Lacan and Pontalis (1967), who point in particular to a passage in Freud's letters to Fließ in which he spoke of memories being subject from time to time to a reordering, to a transcription. Such an understanding can be found, too, in hermeneutical views of psychoanalysis (Kerz-Rühling, 2008) and it corresponds to modern neuroscientific investigations of the processes of memory.

Example of a case: a patient, who from nursery school age onward had been seduced by her father into performing sexual acts, describes that up to the age of ten she had found this perfectly normal. It only then began to feel increasingly problematic. After puberty she developed pronounced symptoms of a chronic post-traumatic stress disorder.

## Denial

*Denial* designates a "primitive" form of *defence* in which a part of reality is excluded from awareness. This means this part of reality is negated and regarded as non-existent. Whereas in repression, which is regarded as the most important mechanism of *defence* in neuroses, reality is acknowledged and only the drive wishes are repressed, that is, become *unconscious*, in *denial* "reality" is "changed". This mechanism is most striking in the schizophrenic psychosis, in which the perception of reality is fundamentally disturbed and in which, for example, paranoid ways of experiencing, obsessions of reference, delusional experiences of being influenced, delusions, and hallucinations all distort perception of reality in grotesque ways. But also in an emotionally unstable personality disorder of the borderline type, *denial* plays a considerable role so that pronounced distortions of reality can develop, particularly in personal relationships.

For example, these patients often keep the good and bad aspects of a person strictly separate from each other because integrating opposites is very hard and tolerating tension often beyond them. Wild idealisations and devaluations are common whereby the corresponding opposite quality of the relationship or person, whether positive or negative, will be completely denied—in the subjective perception of the client they do not exist.

The purpose of *denial*, as with all *defence* mechanisms is to reduce fear. The person will actively ignore perceptions which might be near or beyond what he could handle, which might disturb his inner (psychic) balance and be experienced as traumatic. He does this in order to fend off the rising fear, but this usually offers only temporary and not full protection, and pronounced *denial* has, moreover, considerable negative consequences: it restricts reality testing and leads to rigidity in dealings with other people.

In social work *denial* processes can be the cause of a variety of complications: they can cause completely unrealistic perceptions of the client's own social situation and the state of his relationships and his own behaviour to his children (e.g., violent or neglecting); they can also cause a distorted perception of what is intended by particular measures suggested, idealisation of the relationship to the social worker, and, linked to this, unrealistic expectations of the help offered while totally blanking out the client's own contribution, his own neediness, but also his own resources; and finally they may cause refusal of help combined with simultaneously great need of it.

## Holding function and holding environment

As a part of his theory of a child's early psychic development, Winnicott established the importance of the "good enough mother" and "the good enough environment" for the healthy development of the infant. The *"holding function"* associated with these has not only to satisfy the physiological needs of the infant and protect it from injury but must also be infused with empathy for the psychic needs of the infant, to be *"a live adaption to the infant's needs* [italics in original]. The main thing is the physical holding, and this is the basis of all the more complex aspects of holding, and of environmental provision in general" (Winnicott, 1960, p. 54).

On the basis of this adaption to the needs of the infant, its psychic and concrete "being held", the infant develops a sense of the continuity of being and the ability to experience itself as separate from the mother. Winnicott equates this with the concept of ego strength. He stresses how important this form of motherly care is for the healthy development of the individual as regards a relative freedom from psychotic mechanisms and those on the level of borderline organisation.

Psychoanalytic social work is much concerned with producing and making available a *holding environment*, for example for children who have developed an antisocial tendency or for patients with psychiatric illnesses or who are in a state of social decompensation. When working with clients who turn to them with powerful emotional needs the professionals also need a *holding environment* in the form, for instance, of regular supervision.

## Identification with the aggressor

A child introjects some characteristics of an anxiety object and so assimilates an anxiety experience which he has just undergone. Here, the mechanism of identification or introjection is combined with a second important mechanism. By impersonating the aggressor, assuming his attributes or imitating his aggression, the child transforms himself from the person threatened into the person who makes the threat. (Freud, A., 1936, chap. 9, p. 113)

*Identification with the aggressor* is a *defence* mechanism which primarily serves to deal with perceptions and experiences that flood the ego with fear and threaten to overwhelm it. In doing so it secures the survival of the child's inner world in situations of threat and powerlessness. Particularly in children who have been exposed to abuse, sexual violence, or neglect, this mechanism plays a major role. Among other things it leads to an identification of the victim with aspects of violence and often contributes to the development of feelings of guilt. What can develop is a spiralling of negative experiences of self and in part unconscious self-reproach, feelings of guilt and the person's own violent behaviour which he justifies by projecting the responsibility onto others. The aggressive elements with which the person in question has identified frequently take no further part in his development (but remain in their original form) so that often they are accompanied by very childish ways of thinking and experiencing.

Particularly with violent clients social work is often confronted with identifications of this kind and the cycle of aggression, and also with feelings of inferiority and guilt, which in their turn are warded off with fresh aggression. But also in the work with victims of violence, with their fixation on the violent perpetrator, an understanding of such dynamics is important so that the social worker does not remain trapped in the giving of ineffectual advice or even, via *projective identification*, become infected with aggressive introjections and himself become a "perpetrator".

## Object relations

The term *object relations* refers in the classic Freudian view to the relation of the *subject* (or the *ego* in Freud's terminology, the *self* in later ego psychology) to a love-object that is libidinously cathected. *Object* is to be taken as a psychoanalytical term and often refers to an emotionally cathected person. Cathexis means an investment of affect in an object.

What is meant is not so much the real-world objects, for example, the real parents, but above all the inner objects or object representations, mental representations of the object, whose interplay one can visualise as in a kind of internal theatre in which the different actors appearing on stage would be the inner objects. The inner objects exert decisive influence on how an individual forms his relationships and on his behaviour in terms of affect. Different schools of psychoanalysis emphasise the constitutional, infantile, or the parental, interactional influence on the *object relations* of the child or place the mutual influence of these factors in the centre of their reflections. From the very start of life the intense exchange processes between the inner world of the child and his perception of the outer world mean that inner *objects* are partly shaped through *introjection* of outer *objects*, but that equally the outer *objects* are perceived in the light of inner phantasies and through projection are not always seen realistically.

It is significant, too, that the parents' own inner *objects* influence the interaction between parents and child strongly and that in this way there is a process of passing on of representations and attitudes. While in cognitive psychology the concept of the *object* refers rather to a sensory perception, in the psychoanalytic understanding of the *object relation* an affective and drive component is always present. Klein also produced profound reflections on how integrated or whole *objects* might take shape from so-called part objects in the course of a child's development.

In early development, in the paranoid-schizoid position, *objects* are not experienced as whole *objects* but are split into *part objects* which mainly exist in polarised form, for example, as good, helpful, or bad, persecutory objects. In pathological developments, for instance in borderline personality disorders, this *splitting* can remain susceptible to activation at any time and leads to the *object relations* of these clients being often reduced to a few single functions: the object (the carer) is seen as there only to provide food, to excite, or even to poison the client.

In psychoanalytic social work the metaphor of *inner objects* as "actors" makes a number of the clients' reactions and ways of behaving more understandable, as being determined by their inner worlds. The excessive use of *part objects* in the relationship with the social worker is a frequent problem in the work with clients affected by severe disorders. The social worker is under considerable strain because he does not feel perceived as a whole person but is reduced to just a few of his functions for the client.

## Oedipus complex

The *Oedipus complex* is in Freud's view the central psychic construct which is decisive for psychic health and illness. It is characterised by a triangular relationship that is in full flower somewhere between the ages of four and six: the child loves and desires the parent of the opposite sex and hates the parent of his or her own sex with whom he or she is in contest over the love-object. Freud called this classic *Oedipus complex* structure, that he observed first, the positive *Oedipus complex*. It can, however, appear in many variant forms: in the negative *Oedipus complex*, for instance, the child loves the same-sex parent and hates the other. For a girl the *Oedipus complex* is complicated by the fact that for her development she needs to achieve detachment from the mother, who was her first love-object, providing her with nourishment, whereas the boy, whose case is less complicated, is spared this shift from one object to another. On the other hand, however, boys may unconsciously remain more powerfully tied to the mother whom they hope to find again in later love relationships. If the previous relationship to the mother had been disappointing the necessary change of object demanded of little girls may bind them to her ambivalently, that is, in the hope of yet being able to satisfy previously unsatisfied desires, a condition that is characteristic for depressive and hysterical illnesses.

The overcoming or fading of the *Oedipus complex* is achieved by the child giving up the loved parent as love-object, the first major exercise in renunciation. It is, however, forced on the child by the threatening quality attributed to the rival parent, a result of the child's own destructive impulses towards this parent which it has projected onto him or her. An important step in the fading of the *Oedipus complex* is the child's identification with the real or attributed prohibitions of the competing parent. It leads to the establishment of a coherent inner representation, the superego, composed of various earlier forms. In the place of external, forbidding, and regulating persons the superego increasingly takes over control and guidance of the person. If the *Oedipus complex* is not mastered in this ideal manner there may remain a libidinous, aggressive, or ambivalent clinging to the parental primary objects with resulting neurotic illnesses. The way the parents deal with the child's drive strivings plays a central role in the way the *Oedipus complex* is resolved.

In terms of drive dynamics the *Oedipus complex* shows libidinous and aggressive drive impulses towards the parents. As regards *object relations* the child has to find a specific relation to each parent and to acknowledge the existence of the parents as a sexual couple.

This corresponds to the findings of recent developmental psychology that children between the ages of four and six gain a new understanding of reality, for the distinction between inner and outer, between the *equivalence mode*—or the conviction that a game or object really *is* what the child attributes to it—and the *as-if-mode*, or the ability to realise the "pretend" quality of a doll or a fantasy (Fonagy, Gergely, Jurist & Target, 2002). Important steps in that direction take place—according to present day views—in the early years. In the process of individuation and separation from about the first birthday (Mahler, 1968; Mahler, Pine & Bergman, 1975) the detachment from the maternal primary object is achieved substantially with the help of the father—that is, with the aid of a triangular combination but not yet with sexual connotations in the stricter sense. Melanie Klein spoke of the early *Oedipus complex*, meaning the libidinous and aggressive *cathexis* of the maternal breast as *part object*, a cathexis which is later partly shifted to the paternal penis. So in a way one could call the *Oedipus complex* the maturation of a triangular relationship.

## Projective identification

According to current understanding, *projective identification* is a process of psychic exchange in which one person unconsciously conveys an inner state charged with tension to another person. The concept was created by Melanie Klein (1946) when she was describing what went on between mother and child. In her view *projective identification* is a *defence* mechanism belonging to the paranoid-schizoid position, which is an early stage in development marked by insufficiently integrated anger. The child wards off the anger above all in the form of projection but he fears that his *object*, the person towards whom he feels this anger, is angered by this and will attack him. Paranoid fears develop as a result. In *projective identification* the child projects a psychic state of anger and fear, that is hard to bear, onto the mother who appropriates it in the process of identifying with it. Now she senses this mixture of feelings. *Projective identification* is therefore an intersubjective mechanism—one which, by contrast with other *defence* mechanisms, is not restricted to the subject and which serves to get rid of hard-to-endure and above all aggressively dominated inner states.

Clinically, *projective identification* is seen as occurring in illnesses which are characterised by fixations in the paranoid-schizoid position or regressions to this position.

Signs of *projective identification* in psychoanalytic treatment are for example the analyst's awareness of feelings and inner states that are otherwise alien to him, which he cannot explain to himself on the basis of his own experience, or the preoccupation with a patient continuing beyond the one session into the next sessions, in his spare time or in dreams.

Bion (1962) added to and extended ideas on *projective identification*. In his *container/contained* model for particular psychic processes and states of mind, mother and child form a combination of container and contained. The child uses the mother as a container for undigested or incomprehensible elements (he refers to these as beta elements). If all goes well the mother digests these so as to give them back to the child as alpha elements, that is to say in a form which the child can take in, tolerate, understand, and integrate: a model for psychoanalytic treatment, too.

Ogden (1979) connects these ideas with other *object relation* theories and ego psychology. In the *projective identification* he sees a three-phase process: projection of parts of the self from the self representation to the *object representation* as an inner process; interactional manipulation of an external *object* so that this other person (in social work this would be the social worker) experiences the inner state of the subject; and finally control of these inner states or shared experiencing of them *in* the *object*.

This process leads in the end to something approaching mental-emotional fusion between social worker and client which calls for constant reflection.

In psychoanalytic social work the closeness which often exists between carer and client, the intensity of the relationship, and the kind of disorders the client suffers from can easily induce processes of *projective identification*. They can be perceived in supervision.

## Resistance

In psychoanalysis *resistance* describes a patient's *unconscious* tendencies to work against the psychoanalytic treatment and its continuance. Freud discovered it in the treatment of his hysterical patients, who developed *resistance* to remembering. *Resistance* manifests in many forms as an attitude to the analyst or the treatment, in *acting out* over appointments, in the form of keeping silent, as the inhibition preventing them from expressing certain thoughts that occur to them, in over-amenability in the *defence* against aggressive wish.

In the end any behaviour in the course of a treatment can become a form of *resistance* to the analysis: a *resistance* to remembering, to a deeper insight, or to change.

One special, regularly reappearing form of *resistance* is *transference resistance*. In this, the constellation of attitudes and feelings regarding the analyst which the patient has so far developed serves the purpose in his *unconscious* experience of halting the analysis at the state reached in this *transference* relationship.

For instance, one patient who had often been left alone by her mother continually reproached the analyst with not having enough time for her, and with making the sessions too infrequent and too short. With these reproaches she was trying to prevent herself from remembering and re-experiencing her desperate childhood fears of being alone, thus being arrested in her unhappiness. In the treatment and in social work with adolescents affected by early disorders the *transference resistance* often leads to the doctor or carer being experienced as a malevolent *object* of early childhood and so becoming the target of aggression.

On the other hand the *transference resistance* enables a recognition of the *object* and relationship *representations* and this knowledge can be used in treatment. A frequently occurring form of *resistance* in adolescents with a weak or endangered sense of identity, as can often be the case with antisocial adolescents, is identity *resistance*, opposing any change in their person to prevent their identity being further shaken.

## Splitting

Like practically all psychoanalytic concepts and terms the term *splitting* has undergone developments. Freud spoke of *Spaltung* in a number of contexts: of *Ichspaltung* in psychoses and fetishism, of *Abspaltung*, the *splitting* off of traumatic experiences, and of the *splitting* of consciousness in dissociated states as occur in hysteria.

Melanie Klein (1946) developed her own concept of *splitting* which she saw as being produced by fluctuating states of the self in which the infant is swung back and forth between bliss and extreme fear. She uses *states of the self* as a term for an affective state, an inner state particularly in connection with a dissociated state, but not only in that context.

In Kleinian theory this fear is the child's fear of fragmentation caused by his own delight in destruction. Both states are connected with the maternal breast, at times giving satisfaction and therefore good, at times not satisfying and therefore bad. In this way the child's own destructive impulses are projected outside himself and the self is relieved of them. In the *depressive position* the loving and the aggressive-threatening impulses are combined and integrated.

If no integration is achieved then a tendency to *splitting* and projection of negative impulses into the outer world remains. In this way a view of the world is created that polarises good and bad and it becomes impossible to see positive and negative at the same time in one *object*. Thus idealisation and devaluation stand juxtaposed and irreconcilable. According to Kleinian views as further elaborated by Kernberg (1981) these mechanisms appear particularly in narcissistic and psychotic illnesses.

In their *mentalisation* concept Fonagy, Gergely, Jurist, and Target (2002) see *splitting* tendencies as arising from the experience of neglect or abuse and as leading to a *splitting* of the inner image of the *object*, the parts of which cannot be put together again because of a striving for mental coherence. It is the case that such polarising attitudes can often be observed in clients. Sometimes one and the same person or the client's own person will be idealised one moment and devalued the next. In combination with *projective identification* such *splitting* attributions can lead to real splits in hospital or home group teams.

## Transference

*Transference*, as it was originally understood, is the repetition of feelings felt for an important person in the past or attitudes towards them now directed towards a person in the present. This is associated with a distortion of reality since the true nature of this person is misjudged. In psychoanalytic treatment the *transference* in the so-called *transference* analysis is used to make the *unconscious* and internalised *object relations* and *object representations* of a patient accessible to his conscious mind. A mild positive *transference* is regarded as helpful—for the treatment. Where Freud was of the opinion that the *transference* was exclusively a creation of the patient's *unconscious*, today the prevailing view is that the analyst contributes significantly to its emergence and to the shape it takes. In the case of some illnesses, particularly those of narcissistic or psychotic character, some psychoanalysts are of the opinion that the analyst should actively help to shape if not create the *transference*.

*Transferences* are not restricted to psychoanalytic or psychotherapeutic treatments. They take place in all kinds of contexts. They are approaches to relationships and attempts to shape these relationships to significant others, to whom the person attributes aspects of earlier important *objects*.

*Transferences* trigger corresponding *countertransferences* in the persons at the receiving end. In this way a communication between the *unconscious* of the self and the *object* emerges. In psychoanalytic treatment the *countertransference* is systematically used to decode the patient's *transferences*. On *transference* in psychoanalytic social work see Chapter Ten of this volume.

## Transitional object/potential space

Starting from the observation that infants from the age of three months use some object, usually something soft, for example a piece of cloth, the corner of a blanket, or a soft toy in a particular manner to calm themselves or to go to sleep, Winnicott (1951) developed the concept of the *transitional object*. He characterised these objects as being in an intermediary space between subject and external reality. The use of the *transitional object* enables the infant to accomplish the development of a primary relationship to the mother into a genuine *object* relationship.

The *transitional object* represents, on the one hand, an almost inseparable part of the child's self, and on the other hand it is experienced as the first possession which is not-me and thus contributes crucially to the differentiation between subject and *object*. By reason of its permanent availability it protects the child against his fears of being abandoned. *Transitional objects* and transitional phenomena also play a major role in later life.

As an intermediary area between internal and external reality the whole field of culture, art, religion, science, sport, and similar activities will remain of lifelong significance for a person's ability to enjoy experiences and to enter into relationships. The ability to gain inner access to a transitional space (*potential space*) is essential for every therapeutic relationship in that it enables an element of the playful to mediate between demands of inner drives and rigid orientation to external reality.

Psychoanalytic social work is concerned with the relationship between psychical and external reality and is thus by its very nature at work in this intermediary space. It is important when working with a client to use the *potential space* as an area in which developments are possible. A client's resources are often closely linked to this space and have a chance to develop if it proves possible to set up a better relation between internal and external reality.

## The unconscious

Freud's central discovery and the point of reference for every psycho-analytic theory and practice is the dynamic *unconscious* at work in every human being. Originally Freud conceived of the *unconscious* as being made up of repressed representations of drive, to which the conscious mind has no access but which break through into consciousness in dreams, parapraxis, and symptoms.

Over time the concept became extended so that other psychic proc-esses and contents, namely parts of the superego and of the ego, also came to be conceived of as *unconscious*. In the meantime modern neuro-scientific research has confirmed Freud's finding, which was based on his clinical work, that the far greater part of the psychical apparatus is inaccessible to the conscious mind and is as such *unconscious*.

We have to distinguish, however, between two areas: on the one hand there are automatism skills, such as the command of cultural skills (arithmetic and writing), certain motor capabilities, or the matter-of-course observance of social rules and repertoires of behaviour, which have been acquired through practice and learning and no longer require conscious control; on the other hand, there is the area of *uncon-scious* psychical processes with which psychoanalysis is predominantly concerned: conflictual psychical processes in which, for instance, the opposing interests of drive desires and the demands of conscience appear unresolvable.

Here the desires may be too powerful or the conscience too rigid and judgmental, or even sadistic towards the self. This dynamic *unconscious* is characterised, above all, by the way in which contradictory positions may be maintained unchallenged alongside one another, and by the way in which it functions according to the pleasure principle rather than the reality principle. Thus thinking in the *unconscious* is associative and in this way similar to dream thinking.

One can regard the *unconscious* as a kind of storehouse of memories which is not accessible to conscious exploration and yet has immense influence on our options for action, particularly in emotionally charged contexts.

Symptoms, *parapraxes* (popularly in the singular = a Freudian slip), irrational behaviour, etc. are seen by psychoanalysis as the expression of a compromise between *unconscious* wishes and dispositions on the one hand and the demands of reality on the other.

*Unconscious* communication therefore constantly occurs in everyday life, too, as soon as feelings and desires are involved. In social work it is particularly important because many clients have no way of handling conflicts and contradictions in the central area of their lives other than with the aid of *defence* mechanisms—a process which is linked with a banishing of their desires and needs into the *unconscious*.

Urges of a libidinous or aggressive nature are repressed into the *unconscious* while painful, shaming, hard-to-bear feelings or affects (e.g., fear, depression), but also a person's own abilities, are often denied. Such processes not infrequently stem from difficult biographies with their resultant fixation of childish desires in the *unconscious*. Equally, in the immediacy of the moment, the social worker often reacts unconsciously to the *unconscious* communication of the client.

# REFERENCES

Abraham, K. (1924). Versuch einer Entwicklungsgeschichte der Libido auf Grund der Psychoanalyse seelischer Störungen. In: *Gesammelte Schriften (Volume 2)* (pp. 32–102). Frankfurt/M, Germany: Fischer, 1982.

Aichhorn, A. (1925). *Wayward Youth*. Revised by author. Evanston, IL: Northwest University Press, 1983.

Aichhorn, A. (2006). Die Verwahrlosung einmal anders gesehen (1948). *Kinderanalyse*, *14*: 80–109.

Aichhorn, T. (2006). Vorbemerkungen zu August Aichhorns Vortrag: "Die Verwahrlosung einmal anders gesehen". *Kinderanalyse*, *14*: 63–79.

Allerdings, I. & Staigle, J. (1999). Der Verein für Psychoanalytische Sozialarbeit. 20 Jahre Betreuung von jungen Menschen mit schweren seelischen Handicaps. Zu Gründung, Struktur und Arbeitsbereichen. In: Verein für Psychoanalytische Sozialarbeit (Ed.), *Vom Entstehen Analytischer Räume* (pp. 292–330). [Dokumentation der 9. Fachtagung des Vereins für Psychoanalytische Sozialarbeit im November 1998 in Rottenburg.] Tübingen, Germany: Edition diskord.

Altmeyer, M. & Thomä, H. (2006). *Die Vernetzte Seele. Die Intersubjektive Wende in der Psychoanalyse*. Stuttgart, Germany: Klett-Cotta.

Amthor, R. -C. (2005). Die Geschichte der Berufsausbildung in der Sozialen Arbeit. Kritische Reflexionen zur herkömmlichen Geschichtsschreibung. *Soziale Arbeit*, *2/2005*: 42–50.

Amuser-Burger, H. (1994). Die Herstellung eines Falls. Eine andere Art der Supervision. In: Verein für Psychoanalytische Sozialarbeit (Ed.), *Supervision in der Psychoanalytischen Sozialarbeit* (pp. 121–123). Tübingen, Germany: Edition diskord.

Argelander, H. (1970). Die szenische Funktion des Ichs und ihr Anteil an der Symptom- und Charakterbildung. *Psyche—Zeitschrift für Psychoanalyse, 24*: 325–345.

Bauriedl, T. (2001). Szenische Veränderungsprozesse in der Supervision— Ursache und Wirkmechanismen aus beziehungsanalytischer Sicht. In: B. Oberhoff & U. Beumer (Eds.), *Theorie und Praxis Psychoanalytischer Supervision* (pp. 27–48). Münster, Germany: Votum Verlag.

Becker, H. (Ed.) (1995a). *Psychoanalytische Teamsupervision.* Göttingen, Germany: Vandenhoeck & Ruprecht.

Becker, H. (1995b). Angewandte Psychoanalyse in der Teamsupervision als Forschungsansatz. Zur Ethnopsychoanalyse psychiatrischer Institutionen. In: H. Becker (Ed.), *Psychoanalytische Teamsupervision* (pp. 179–228). Göttingen, Germany: Vandenhoeck & Ruprecht.

Becker, H. & Nedelmann, C. (Eds.) (1987). Psychoanalytische Sozialarbeit mit psychotischen Kindern und Jugendlichen. *Psychosozial, 10*(32).

Becker, S. (Ed.) (1991). *Psychose und Grenze. Zur Endlichen und Unendlichen Psychoanalytischen Sozialarbeit mit Psychotischen Kindern, Jugendlichen, jungen Erwachsenen und Ihren Familien.* Tübingen, Germany: Edition diskord.

Belardi, N. (1998). *Supervision. Eine Einführung für Soziale Berufe.* Freiburg i. Br., Germany: Lambertus.

Bernfeld, S. (1925). *Sisyphus or the Limits of Education.* F. Lilge (Trans.). Berkeley, CA: University of California Press, 1973.

Besemer, C. (1993). *Mediation. Vermittlung in Konflikten* (12th edition). Königsfeld, Germany: Stiftung Gewaltfreies Leben, 2007.

Bettelheim, B. (1950). *Love Is Not Enough: The Treatment of Emotionally Disturbed Children.* Glencoe, IL: Free Press.

Bettelheim, B. (1967). *The Empty Fortress: Infantile Autism and the Birth of the Self.* New York: Free Press.

Bettelheim, B. (1976). *The Uses of Enchantment.* New York: Alfred A. Knopf.

Bielefelder Arbeitsgruppe 8 (Ed.) (2008). Soziale Arbeit in Gesellschaft. Wiesbaden, Germany: VS Verlag für Sozialwissenschaften.

Bion, W. R. (1957). Differentiation of the psychotic from the non-psychotic personalities. *International Journal of Psychoanalysis, 38*: 266–275.

Bion, W. R. (1962a). *Learning from Experience.* London: Heinemann [reprinted London: Karnac, reprinted in *Seven Servants* (Bion, 1977e)].

Bion, W. R. (1962b). The psycho-analytic study of thinking. *International Journal of Psychoanalysis, 43*: 306–310.

Bion, W. R. (1984). *Second Thoughts. Selected Papers on Psychoanalysis.* London: Karnac.

Birgmeier, B. R. (2005). Sozialpädagogik als Handlungswissenschaft. Wissenschaftstheoretische Fragen und Antworten einer handlungstheoretisch fundierten Sozialpädagogik. *Sozialmagazin, 30*(5): 38–49.

Bleger, J. (1966). Die Psychoanalyse des psychoanalytischen Rahmens. *Forum der Psychoanalyse, 9*(1993): 268–280.

Bleiberg, E. (2001). *Treating Personality Disorders in Children and Adolescents*. New York: Guilford.

Blos, P. (1973). *Adoleszenz*. Stuttgart, Germany: Klett-Cotta, 1979.

Bohleber, W. (1999). Psychoanalyse, Adoleszenz und das Problem der Identität. *Psyche—Zeitschrift für Psychoanalyse, 53*: 507–529.

Bohleber, W. (2008). Einige Probleme psychoanalytischer Traumatheorie. In: M. Leuzinger-Bohleber, G. Roth, & A. Buchheim (Eds.), *Psychoanalyse, Neurobiologie, Trauma* (pp. 45–54). Stuttgart, Germany: Schattauer.

Bosch, S. & Feuling, M. (1997). Vom willkürlichen anderen zum Gesetz des Sozialen. In: Verein für Psychoanalytische Sozialarbeit (Ed.), *Vom Umgehen mit Aggressivität. Zur Bewältigung von Psychotischer Angst, Depression und Agierter Aggression* (pp. 23–46). [Dokumentation der 8. Fachtagung des Vereins für Psychoanalytische Sozialarbeit im November 1996 in Rottenburg.] Tübingen, Germany: Edition diskord.

Bruns, G. (1989). Das vorbildliche Lehrerkind. Zur Soziogenese einer Familienneurose. *Forum der Psychoanalyse, 5*: 300–318.

Bruns, G. (1991). Vorbildlichkeit als Auftrag. Selbstidealisierung und neurotische Störungen in Lehrerfamilien. In: C. Büttner & U. Finger-Trescher (Eds.), *Psychoanalyse und Schulische Konflikte* (pp. 93–109). Mainz, Germany: Grünewald.

Bruns, G. (1994). Warum Lehrer den Buckel hinhalten. Psychoanalytische Bemerkungen zu Lust, Angst und Moral in der Schule. *Pädagogik, 46*(6): 21–25.

Bruns, G. (1995). Soziale Vernetzung—ein Parameter in der psychoanalytischen Behandlung psychotischer Patienten. *Forum der Psychoanalyse, 11*: 84–94.

Bruns, G. (1996). Überlegungen zu einer Psychopathologie der ästhetischen Rezeption. In: H. Haselbeck, M. Heuser, H. Hinterhuber, & W. Pöldinger (Eds.), *Kränkung, Angst und Kreativität* (pp. 216–224). Innsbruck, Austria: Verlag Integrative Psychiatrie.

Bruns, G. (1998). Einige sozialpsychiatrische Konzepte und ihre Grenzen aus psychoanalytischer Sicht. *Sozialpsychiatrische Informationen, 28*(2): 6–15.

Bruns, G. (1999). Analytischer Raum—Psychose—Institution. In: Verein für Psychoanalytische Sozialarbeit (Ed.), *Vom Entstehen Analytischer Räume* (pp. 235–247). Tübingen, Germany: Edition diskord.

Bruns, G. (2006). Was ist psychoanalytische Sozialarbeit? *Kinderanalyse, 14*: 4–20.

Budde, W. & Früchtel, F. (2005). Fall und Feld. Oder was in der sozialraumorientierten Fallarbeit mit Netzwerken zu machen ist. Das Beispiel Eco-Mapping und Genogrammarbeit. *Sozialmagazin, 30*(6): 14–23.

Büttner, C. & Finger-Trescher, U. (Eds.) (1991). *Psychoanalyse und Schulische Konflikte*. Mainz, Germany: Grünewald.

Büttner, C., Finger-Trescher, U. & Scherpner, M. (Eds.) (1990). *Psychoanalyse und Soziale Arbeit*. Mainz, Germany: Grünewald.

Butterwegge, C. (2005). Wohlfahrtsstaat und Soziale Arbeit im Zeichen der Globalisierung. In: K. Störch (Ed.), *Soziale Arbeit in der Krise* (pp. 12–38). Hamburg, Germany: VSA-Verlag.

Chassé, K. A. & von Wensierski, H. -J. (1999). *Praxisfelder der Sozialen Arbeit* (3rd edition). Weinheim, Germany: Juventa, 2004.

Denner, S. (2008). *Soziale Arbeit mit psychisch kranken Kindern und Jugendlichen*. Stuttgart, Germany: Kohlhammer.

Deutsch, H. (1926). Okkulte Vorgänge während der Psychoanalyse. *Imago, 12*: 418–433.

Deutsche Gesellschaft für Sozialarbeit (2005). Kerncurriculum Soziale Arbeit/Sozialarbeitswissenschaft für Bachelor- und Masterstudiengänge in Sozialer Arbeit. *Sozialmagazin, 30*(4): 15–23.

Dornes, M. (2000). *Die Emotionale Welt des Kindes*. Frankfurt/M., Germany: Fischer.

Dornes, M. (2006). *Die Seele des Kindes. Entstehung und Entwicklung*. Frankfurt/M., Germany: Fischer.

du Bois, R. & Gunter, M. (2000). Psychoanalytisch orientierte Behandlung schwerer juveniler Psychosen im stationären Setting. *Forum der Psychoanalyse, 16*: 315–330.

Duss-von Werdt, J. (2005). *Homo Mediator. Geschichte und Menschenbild der Mediation*. Stuttgart, Germany: Klett-Cotta.

Engelbrecht, H. (1990). Die Inszenierung der psychoanalytischen Situation in der Supervision. *Psyche—Zeitschrift für Psychoanalyse, 44*: 675–688.

Engelke, E., Maier, K., Steinert, E., Borrmann, S. & Spatschek, C. (2007). *Forschung für die Praxis. Zum Gegenwärtigen Stand der Sozialarbeitsforschung*. Freiburg i. Br., Germany: Lambertus.

Erler, M. (1993). *Soziale Arbeit. Ein Lehr- und Arbeitsbuch zu Geschichte, Aufgaben und Theorie* (6th edition). Weinheim: Juventa, 2007.

Federn, E. (1985). Das Verhältnis von Psychoanalyse und Sozialarbeit in historischer und prinzipieller Sicht. In: J. C. Aigner (Ed.), *Sozialarbeit und Psychoanalyse. Chancen und Probleme in der Praktischen Arbeit* (pp. 13–30). Graz, Austria: Verband der wissenschaftlichen Gesellschaften Österreichs.

Federn, E. (1994). Supervision in der psychoanalytischen Sozialarbeit. In: Verein für psychoanalytische Sozialarbeit (Ed.), *Supervision in der Psychoanalytischen Sozialarbeit* (pp. 12–20). Tübingen, Germany: Edition diskord.

Ferenczi, S. & Rank, O. (1924). *The Development of Psychoanalysis*. New York: Nervous and Mental Disease Publishing, 1925.

Feuling, M. (1997). Die Frage nach dem Gesetz des Sozialen. Eine Fallgeschichte. In: *Arbeitshefte Kinderpsychoanalyse (Volume 24): Verbot, Gesetz und Übertretung—Überlegungen zum Historischen Ort von Erziehungsnotständen* (pp. 61–81). Kassel, Germany, 1997.

Feuling, M. (2006). Verharren in Sackgassen. Aspekte der Dialektik von Herr und Knecht in der psychoanalytischen Sozialarbeit. *Kinderanalyse*, 14: 21–43.

Finger-Trescher, U. (2001). Psychoanalytische Sozialarbeit. In: H. -U. Otto & H. Thiersch (Eds.), *Handbuch Sozialarbeit Sozialpädagogik* (pp. 1454–1461). Neuwied, Germany: Luchterhand.

Fonagy, P. (2001). *Attachment Theory and Psychoanalysis*. New York: Other.

Fonagy, P., Gergely, G., Jurist, E. L. & Target, M. (2002). *Affect Regulation, Mentalization, and the Development of the Self*. New York: Other.

Foulkes, S. H. (1975). *Praxis der Gruppenanalytischen Psychotherapie*. München, Germany: Reinhardt, 1978.

Freud, A. (1936). *The Writings of Anna Freud (Volume II)* (revised edition). New York: International Universities Press, 1966, chap. 9, p. 113.

Freud, S. (1895b). On the grounds for detaching a particular syndrome from neurasthenia under the description "anxiety neurosis". *S. E.*, *3*. London: Hogarth, pp. 85–115.

Freud, S. (1900a). *The Interpretation of Dreams*. *S. E.*, *4–5*. London: Hogarth, pp. IX–627.

Freud, S. (1905d). Three essays on the theory of sexuality. *S. E.*, *7*. London: Hogarth, pp. 123–246.

Freud, S. (1905e). Fragment of an analysis of a case of hysteria. *S. E.*, *7*. London: Hogarth, pp. 1–122.

Freud, S. (1908e). Creative writers and day-dreaming. *S. E.*, *9*. London: Hogarth, pp. 141–154.

Freud, S. (1909d). Notes upon a case of obsessional neurosis. *S. E.*, *10*. London: Hogarth, pp. 151–318.

Freud, S. (1910d). The future prospects of psycho-analytic therapy. *S. E.*, *11*. London: Hogarth, pp. 139–152.

Freud, S. (1912b). The dynamics of transference. *S. E.*, *12*. London: Hogarth, pp. 97–108.

Freud, S. (1914f). Some reflections on schoolboy psychology. *S. E.*, *13*. London: Hogarth, pp. 239–244.

Freud, S. (1914g). Remembering, repeating and working-through (further recommendations on the technique of psycho-analysis, II). *S. E.*, *12*. London: Hogarth, pp. 145–156.

Freud, S. (1915a). Observations on transference-love (further recommendations on the technique of psycho-analysis, III). *S. E., 12*. London: Hogarth, pp. 157–171.

Freud, S. (1915c). Instincts and their vicissitudes. *S. E., 14*. London: Hogarth, pp. 109–140.

Freud, S. (1916–17). Introductory lectures on psycho-analysis. *S. E., 15–16*. London: Hogarth.

Freud, S. (1919a). Lines of advance in psycho-analytic therapy. *S. E., 17*. London: Hogarth, pp. 157–168.

Freud, S. (1920g). Beyond the Pleasure Principle. *S. E., 18*. London: Hogarth, pp. 1–64.

Freud, S. (1923b). The Ego and the Id. *S. E., 19*. London: Hogarth, pp. 1–66.

Freud, S. (1925f). Preface to Aichhorn's *Wayward Youth. S. E., 19*. London: Hogarth, pp. 271–276.

Freud, S. (1930a). Civilization and Its Discontents. *S. E., 21*. London: Hogarth, pp. 57–146.

Freud, S. (1937c). Analysis Terminable and Interminable. *S. E., 23*. London: Hogarth, pp. 209–254.

Freud, S. & Breuer, J. (1895d). Studies on hysteria. *S. E., 2*.

Früchtel, F., Budde, W. & Cyprian, G. (2007). *Sozialer Raum und Soziale Arbeit. Fieldbook: Methoden und Techniken.* Wiesbaden, Germany: VS Verlag für Sozialwissenschaften.

Füchtner, H. (1978). Psychoanalytische Pädagogik. Über das Verschwinden einer Wissenschaft und die Folgen. *Psyche—Zeitschrift für Psychoanalyse, 32*: 193–210.

Fürstenau, P. (1964). Zur Psychoanalyse der Schule als Institution. In: W. F. Haug & C. Müller-Wirth (Eds.), *Das Argument 29—Schule und Erziehung I* (pp. 65–78). Berlin: Argument-Verlag.

Galuske, M. (1998). *Methoden der Sozialen Arbeit* (7th edition). Weinheim, Germany: Juventa, 2007.

Geißler, P. & Rückert, K. (2000). *Mediation—die Neue Streitkultur.* Gießen, Germany: Psychosozial.

Gill, M. M. (1984). Transference: A change in conception or only in emphasis? A response. *Psychoanalytic Inquiry, 4*: 489–523.

Götz, M. & Schäfer, C. D. (2008). *Mediation im Gemeinwesen.* Baltmannsweiler, Germany: Schneider Hohengehren.

Grohmann, F., Gschwender, A. & Schmidt, O. (1993). Fenster zum Rahmen. Begegnungen auf-einander-zu im Therapeutischen Heim Rottenburg. In: Verein für Psychoanalytische Sozialarbeit (Ed.), *Innere Orte—Äußere Orte* (pp. 87–125). Tübingen, Germany: Edition diskord.

Gunter, M. (1994). Psychoanalytische Supervision in der Behandlung und Betreuung chronisch psychotischer und autistisch psychotischer junger Erwachsener. In: Verein für Psychoanalytische Sozialarbeit (Ed.),

*Supervision in der Psychoanalytischen Sozialarbeit* (pp. 178–187). Tübingen, Germany: Edition diskord.

Gunter, M. (2000). Zersplitterung und Containment. Die stationäre Behandlung jugendlicher Psychosen. *Kinderanalyse, 8*: 266–288.

Gunter, M. (2006a). "Leicht beieinander wohnen die Gedanken, doch hart im Raume stoßen sich die Sachen." (Wallenstein)—Die Quadratur des Kreises in der psychoanalytischen Sozialarbeit: Das Unbewusste, der Kühlschrank, das Spiel und die Werkstatt. *Kinderanalyse, 14*: 44–62.

Gunter, M. (2006b): Die Insel, die es nicht gibt. Leben im Niemandsland zwischen äußerer Realität und inneren Objekten. In: B. Nissen (Ed.), *Autistische Phänomene in psychoanalytischen Behandlungen* (pp. 307–322). Gießen, Germany: Psychosozial.

Gunter, M. (2008): "Ach Papa, du bist so peinlich ...". Schamabwehr, Affektkontrolle und narzisstische Stabilität in der Adoleszenzentwicklung. *Psyche—Zeitschrift für Psychoanalyse, 62*: 887–904.

Hartmann, H. (1948). Comments on the psychoanalytic theory of instinctual drives. *Psychoanalytic Quarterly, 17*: 368–388.

Hartmann, H. (1950). Comments on the psychoanalytic theory of the ego. *Psychoanalytic Study of the Child, 5*: 74–96.

Hartmann, H. (1958). Ego psychology and the problem of adaptation. D. Rapaport (Trans.). New York: International Universities Press.

Haynes, J. (2004). Das Aushandeln von Grenzen: Mediation bei einem Fall von sexueller Belästigung am Arbeitsplatz. In: J. M. Haynes, A. Mecke, R. Bastine, & L. S. Fong., *Mediation—vom Konflikt zur Lösung* (pp. 12–171). Stuttgart, Germany: Klett-Cotta.

Hechler, O. (2005). *Psychoanalytische Supervision sozialpädagogischer Praxis. Eine Empirische Untersuchung über die Arbeitsweise fallzentrierter Teamsupervision.* Frankfurt/M., Germany: Brandes & Apsel.

Heimann, P. (1950). On counter-transference. *International Journal of Psychoanalysis, 31*: 81–84.

Heite, C. (2008). *Soziale Arbeit im Kampf um Anerkennung. Professionstheoretische Perspektiven.* Weinheim, Germany: Juventa.

Herold, H. & Weiß, H. (2008). Übertragung. In: W. Mertens & B. Waldvogel (Eds.), *Handbuch psychoanalytischer Grundbegriffe* (3rd edition) (pp. 799–811). Stuttgart: Kohlhammer.

Herzog, B. (2007). *Unsere Schule streitet mit Gewinn. Alltagskonflikte und ihre Mediation.* Göttingen, Germany: Vandenhoeck & Ruprecht.

Hochheimer, W. (1959). Zur Tiefenpsychologie des pädagogischen Feldes. In: U. Derbolav & H. Roth (Eds.), *Psychologie und Pädagogik: Neue Forschungen und Ergebnisse* (pp. 207–238). Heidelberg, Germany: Quelle & Meyer.

Hoffman, I. Z. (1991). Discussion: Toward a social-constructivist view of the psychoanalytic situation. *Psychoanalytic Dialogues, 1*: 74–105.

220    REFERENCES

220    REFERENCES

Hoffman, I. Z. (1998). *Ritual and spontaneity in the psychoanalytic process. A dialectical-constructivist view.* Hillsdale, NJ: Analytic Press.

Hondrich, K. O. (1997). Latente und manifeste Sozialität. Anregungen aus der Psychoanalyse für eine Sozioanalyse. In: P. Kutter (Ed.), *Psychoanalyse interdisziplinär* (pp. 69–95). Frankfurt/M., Germany: Suhrkamp.

Honneth, A. (1992). *Kampf um Anerkennung. Zur Moralischen Grammatik Sozialer Konflikte.* Frankfurt/M., Germany: Suhrkamp.

Jacobson, E. (1964). *Das Selbst und die Welt der Objekte.* Frankfurt/M., Germany: Suhrkamp, 1978.

Kaufhold, R. (2001). *Bettelheim, Ekstein, Federn: Impulse für die Psychoanalytisch-pädagogische Bewegung.* Gießen, Germany: Psychosozial-Verlag.

Kernberg, O. F. (1981). *Objektbeziehungen und die Praxis der Psychoanalyse.* Stuttgart, Germany: Klett-Cotta.

Kerz-Rühling, I. (1993). Nachträglichkeit. *Psyche—Zeitschrift für Psychoanalyse, 47*: 911–933.

Kerz-Rühling, I. (2008). Nachträglichkeit. In: W. Mertens & B. Waldvogel (Eds.), *Handbuch Psychoanalytischer Grundbegriffe* (3rd edition). Stuttgart, Germany: Kohlhammer.

Klawe, W. (2005). Subjektorientierte Netzwerkarbeit zwischen Fallbezug und Sozialraum. *Sozialmagazin, 30*(6): 24–32.

Klein, M. (1932). *The Psycho-Analysis of Children.* London: Hogarth, The International Psycho-Analytical Library, 22.

Klein, M. (1946). Notes on some schizoid mechanisms. *International Journal of Psychoanalysis, 27*: 99–110.

Kleve, H. (2005). Postmoderne Sozialarbeit und Sozialstaatstransformation. Fragen und Antworten aus einer ambivalenzreflexiven Perspektive. *Sozialmagazin, 30*(2): 34–42.

Klüwer, R. (1983). Agieren und Mitagieren. *Psyche—Zeitschrift für Psychoanalyse, 37*: 828–840.

Kohut, H. (1971). *The Analysis of the Self. A Systematic Approach to the Psychoanalytic Treatment of Narcissistic Personality Disorders.* New York: International Universities Press.

Körner, J. (1980). Über das Verhältnis von Psychoanalyse und Pädagogik. *Psyche—Zeitschrift für Psychoanalyse, 34*: 769–789.

Kraft, E. & Perner, A. (1997). Vom Objekt der Betreuung zum Subjekt des Wunsches. Über psychoanalytische Sozialarbeit mit einer 18-jährigen Frau. In: W. Datler, U. Finger-Trescher, & C. Büttner (Eds.), *Jahrbuch für Psychoanalytische Pädagogik* (pp. 10–26). Gießen, Germany: Psychosozial-Verlag.

Kraus, M. H. (2005). *Mediation—wie geht denn das? Ein Praxis-Handbuch für Außergerichtliche Streitbeilegung.* Paderborn, Germany: Junfermann.

Krüger, R. & Zimmermann, G. (2005). Gemeinwesenorientierung, Sozialräume, das Budget und der Verlust von Fortschrittlichkeit in der

Jugendhilfe. In: K. Störch (Ed.), *Soziale Arbeit in der Krise* (pp. 248–258). Hamburg, Germany: VSA-Verlag.

Kruse, J. (2005). Soziale Netzwerkarbeit im Spiegel gegenwärtiger Diskurse. *Sozialmagazin, 30*(6): 36–45.

Kuhles, H. (2007). *Autismus bei Kindern und Jugendlichen. Wege aus der Isolation.* Oldenburg, Germany: Paulo Freire Verlag.

Kutter, P. (2000). Spiegelungen und Übertragungen in der Supervision. In: H. Pühl (Ed.), *Handbuch der Supervision 2* (pp. 41–53). Berlin: Edition Marhold.

Laplanche, J. & Pontalis, J. -B. (1967). *Das Vokabular der Psychoanalyse Vol. 1 & 2.* Frankfurt/M., Germany: Suhrkamp, 1973.

Laufer, M. & Laufer, M. E. (1989). *Adoleszenz und Entwicklungskrise.* Stuttgart, Germany: Klett-Cotta.

Lazar, R. A. (2002). Bions Modell "Container-Contained" und seine Implikationen für die Praxis der Supervision. In: H. Pühl (Ed.), *Supervision— Aspekte organisationeller Beratung* (pp. 165–178). Berlin: Ulrich Leutner Verlag.

Leuzinger-Bohleber, M. (2009). *Frühe Kindheit als Schicksal? Trauma, Embodiment, Soziale Desintegration. Psychoanalytische Perspektiven.* Stuttgart, Germany: Kohlhammer.

Loch, W. (1995). *Theorie und Praxis von Balint-Gruppen. Gesammelte Aufsätze.* Tübingen, Germany: Edition diskord.

Lorenzer, A. (1970). *Sprachzerstörung und Rekonstruktion.* Frankfurt/M., Germany: Suhrkamp.

Lorenzer, A. (1983). Sprache, Lebenspraxis und szenisches Verstehen in der psychoanalytischen Therapie. *Psyche—Zeitschrift für Psychoanalyse, 37*: 97–115.

Lützenkirchen, A. (2008). *Depression im Alter. Soziale Arbeit und Versorgungsstruktur.* Frankfurt/M., Germany: Mabuse-Verlag.

Maas, M. (2004). Der Prophet im eigenen Lande ... . Ernst Federns langer Weg für die psychoanalytische Sozialarbeit. *Kinderanalyse, 12*: 272–287.

Mack-Brunswick, R. (1928). Die Analyse eines Eifersuchtswahnes. *Internationale Zeitschrift für Psychoanalyse, 14*: 458–508.

Mahler, M. S. (1968). *Symbiose und Individuation. Psychosen im Frühen Kindesalter* (4th edition). Stuttgart, Germany: Klett-Cotta.

Mahler, M. S., Pine, F. & Bergman, A. (1975). *Die Psychische Geburt des Menschen.* Frankfurt/M., Germany: Fischer, 1980.

Mäurer, U. (2006). Dokumentation über die Abläufe und Zusammenhänge im Todesfall Kevin K. http://www.vafk.de/bremen/kevin-web/zusammenfassung_bericht_maeurer_20061031.pdf

May, M. (2008). *Aktuelle Theoriediskurse sozialer Arbeit.* Wiesbaden, Germany: VS Verlag für Sozialwissenschaften.

Mentzos, S. (1988). *Interpersonelle und institutionalisierte Abwehr.* Frankfurt/M., Germany: Suhrkamp.

Metzger, T. (2000). Chancen der ehrenamtlichen Mediation. Ein Vergleich der Gemeinwesenmediation in Deutschland, England und den USA. In: P. Geißler & K. Rückert (Eds.), *Mediation—die Neue Streitkultur* (pp. 237–250). Gießen, Germany: Psychosozial Verlag.

Möller, H. (2001). *Was ist Gute Supervision? Grundlagen—Merkmale—Methoden.* Stuttgart, Germany: Klett-Cotta.

Möller, M. L. (1977). Self and object in countertransference. *International Journal of Psychoanalysis, 58*: 365–374.

Nonnenmann, H. (2003). Geteilte Angst ist halbe Angst? Aspekte stationärer Arbeit mit früh strukturell gestörten Jugendlichen und jungen Erwachsenen. In: Verein für Psychoanalytische Sozialarbeit (Ed.), *Angst. Überwältigung—Bewältigung* (pp. 130–147). Tübingen, Germany: Edition diskord.

Ogden, T. H. (1979). On projective identification. *International Journal of Psychoanalysis, 60*: 357–379.

Ogden, T. H. (1994). The concept of interpretive action. *Psychoanalytic Quarterly, 63*: 219–245.

Ortmann, K. & Röh, D. (2008). *Klinische Sozialarbeit. Konzepte—Praxis—Perspektiven.* Freibug i.Br., Germany: Lambertus.

Pietzcker, C. (1992). *Lesend interpretieren. Zur psychoanalytischen Deutung literarischer Texte.* Würzburg, Germany: Königshausen & Neumann.

Pollack, T. (1995). Zur Methodik und Technik psychoanalytischer Teamsupervision. In: H. Becker (Ed.), *Psychoanalytische Teamsupervision* (pp. 51–78). Göttingen, Germany: Vandenhoeck & Ruprecht.

Pühl, H. (Ed.) (1999). *Supervision und Organisationsentwicklung. Handbuch 3.* Opladen, Germany: Leske und Budrich.

Pühl, H. (Ed.) (2000). *Handbuch der Supervision 2.* Berlin: Edition Marhold.

Pühl, H. (Ed.) (2003). *Mediation in Organisationen.* Berlin: Leutner.

Pühl, H. (2004). Versuch, die Mediation in einer Organisation aus psychoanalytisch-systemischer Sicht zu betrachten. In: Triangel-Institut (Ed.), *Brücken und Tücken psychoanalytisch-systemischer Beratung* (pp. 106–117). Berlin: Leutner.

Racker, H. (1959). *Übertragung und Gegenübertragung.* München, Germany: Reinhardt.

Redl, F. & Wineman, D. (1951). *Children Who Hate: The Disorganization and Breakdown of Behavior Controls,* Glencoe, IL: Free Press.

Roudinesco, E. & Plon, M. (1997). *Wörterbuch der Psychoanalyse.* Vienna: Springer, 2004.

Sandler, J. (1976). Gegenübertragung und die Bereitschaft zur Rollenübernahme. *Psyche—Zeitschrift für Psychoanalyse, 30*: 297–305.

Schaub, H. -A. (2007). *Klinische Sozialarbeit. Ausgewählte Theorien, Methoden und Arbeitsfelder in Praxis und Forschung.* Göttingen, Germany: V&R unipress.

Schilling, J. (2005). *Soziale Arbeit. Geschichte—Theorie—Profession.* München, Germany: Reinhardt.

Schlittmaier, A. (2005). Wissenschaftstheoretische Elemente einer Praxiswissenschaft. Überlegungen zur Theoriebildung im Rahmen einer Sozialarbeitswissenschaft. *Sozialmagazin, 30*(3): 26–30.

Schmidt, O. (1995). "Ich glaub' ich hab' ein Loch in der Seele"—Bruchstücke (aus) der Begegnung mit einem psychotischen Jugendlichen im Therapeutischen Heim. In: Verein für Psychoanalytische Sozialarbeit (Ed.), *Fragen zur Ethik und Technik Psychoanalytischer Sozialarbeit* (pp. 172–204). Tübingen, Germany: Edition diskord.

Schulz, O. (2008). Ein klärender Spaziergang im Land der Begriffe zwischen Gemeinwesen-, Stadtteil- und Nachbarschaftsmediation. In: M. Götz & C. D. Schäfer (Eds.), *Mediation im Gemeinwesen* (pp. 84–105). Baltmannsweiler, Germany: Schneider Hohengehren.

Searles, H. F. (1963). Übertragungspsychosen bei der Psychotherapie von chronischer Schizophrenie. In: *Der psychoanalytische Beitrag zur Schizophrenieforschung* (pp. 205–258). München, Germany: Kindler, 1974.

Segal, H. (1957). Notes on symbol formation. *International Journal of Psychoanalysis, 38*: 391–397.

Sorg, R. (2005). Soziale Arbeit 2004. In: K. Störch, K. (Ed.), *Soziale Arbeit in der Krise* (pp. 39–63). Hamburg, Germany: VSA-Verlag.

Spatschek, C. (2005). Soziale Arbeit im neoliberalen Kontext. Perspektiven für eine professionelle Modernisierung. *Soziale Arbeit, 3*(2005): 94–103.

Speck, K. (2007). *Schulsozialarbeit.* München, Germany: Reinhardt.

Spence, D. P. (1982). *Narrative Truth and Historical Truth. Meaning and Interpretation in Psychoanalysis.* New York: W. W. Norton.

Steinhardt, K. (2005). *Psychoanalytisch orientierte Supervision. Auf dem Weg zu einer Profession?* Gießen, Germany: Psychosozial Verlag.

Stemmer-Lück, M. (2004). *Beziehungsräume in der Sozialen Arbeit.* Stuttgart, Germany: Kohlhammer.

Sterba, R. (1934). Das Schicksal des Ichs im therapeutischen Verfahren. *Internationale Zeitschrift für Psychoanalyse, 20*: 66–73.

Stern, D. N. (1992). *Die Lebenserfahrung des Säuglings.* Stuttgart, Germany: Klett-Cotta.

Stern, D. N. (1998). *Die Mutterschaftskonstellation. Eine vergleichende Darstellung der verschiedenen Formen der Mutter-Kind-Psychotherapie.* Stuttgart, Germany: Klett-Cotta.

Stone, L. (1961). *Die psychoanalytische Situation.* Frankfurt/M., Germany: Fischer, 1973.

Streeck-Fischer, A. (1994). Entwicklungslinien der Adoleszenz. Narzissmus und Übergangsphänomene. *Psyche—Zeitschrift für Psychoanalyse, 48*: 509–528.

Streeck-Fischer, A. (Ed.) (2004). *Adoleszenz—Bindung—Destruktivität*. Stuttgart, Germany: Klett-Cotta.

Trescher, H. -G. (1990). *Theorie und Praxis der psychoanalytischen Pädagogik*. Mainz, Germany: Grünewald.

Tustin, F. (1990). *The Protective Shell in Children and Adults*. London: Karnac.

Verein für Psychoanalytische Sozialarbeit (Ed.) (1993). *Innere Orte—Äußere Orte. Die Bildung psychischer Strukturen bei Ich-strukturell gestörten Menschen*. Tübingen, Germany: Edition diskord.

Verein für Psychoanalytische Sozialarbeit (Ed.) (1994). *Supervision in der Psychoanalytischen Sozialarbeit*. Tübingen, Germany: Edition diskord.

Verein für Psychoanalytische Sozialarbeit (Ed.) (1997). *Vom Umgehen mit Aggressivität. Zur Bewältigung von psychotischer Angst, Depression und agierter Aggression*. Tübingen, Germany: Edition diskord.

Verein für Psychoanalytische Sozialarbeit (Ed.) (2000). *Afrika ist um die Ecke. Psychoanalytische Sozialarbeit in der "gesprengten Institution" Hagenwört*. Tübingen, Germany: Edition diskord.

Wallerstein, R. S. (1988). One psychoanalysis or many? *International Journal of Psychoanalysis, 69*: 5–22.

Weber, M. (1905). Die protestantische Ethik und der Geist des Kapitalismus. In: *Die protestantische Ethik I* (pp. 27–277). Hamburg: Siebenstern, 1973.

Weiß, R. (1936). Psychoanalyse und Schule. Ein Sammelbericht. *Zeitschrift für Psychoanalytische Pädagogik, 10*: 321–336.

Werder, L. & von Wolff, R. (Eds.) (1974). *Siegfried Bernfeld. Antiautoritäre Erziehung und Psychoanalyse. Ausgewählte Schriften Volumes 1–3*. Frankfurt/M., Germany: Ullstein.

Winnicott, D. W. (1951). Transitional objects and transitional phenomena - a study of the first not-me possession. *International Journal of Psychoanalysis, 34*: 89–97.

Winnicott, D. W. (1960). The theory of the parent-infant relationship. In: D. W. Winnicott, *The Maturational Process and the Facilitating Environment* (p. 54). London: Hogarth, 1965.

Winnicott, D. W. (1971a). *Playing and Reality*. London: Tavistock, 1971.

Winnicott, D. W. (1971b). *Therapeutic Consultations in Child Psychiatry*. London: Hogarth.

Winnicott, D. W. (1984). *Deprivation and Delinquency*. London: Tavistock.

Winter, F. (Ed.) (2004). *Der Täter-Opfer-Ausgleich und die Vision von einer "heilenden" Gerechtigkeit*. Worpswede, Germany: Amberg-Verlag.

# INDEX